for Danny,
+ Brigitte
How does your
wild
body
want to move?....

♡ Ruthie F.

STACK YOUR BONES

100 simple lessons for realigning your body and moving with ease

RUTHIE FRASER

Foreword by Cyndi Lee

THE EXPERIMENT

NEW YORK

To Myles Orion and Uncle Bobby

STACK YOUR BONES: *100 Simple Lessons for Realigning Your Body and Moving with Ease*
Copyright © 2017 by Ruthie Fraser
Foreword © 2017 by Cyndi Lee
Illustrations copyright © 2017 by Ruthie Fraser
Photographs copyright © 2017 by Evan Sklar

Page 241 constitutes a continuation of the copyright page.

The Experiment, LLC, 220 East 23rd Street, Suite 301, New York, NY 10010-4674
theexperimentpublishing.com

This book contains the opinions and ideas of its author. It is intended to provide helpful and informative material on the subjects addressed in the book. It is sold with the understanding that the author and publisher are not engaged in rendering medical, health, or any other kind of personal professional services in the book. The author and publisher specifically disclaim all responsibility for any liability, loss, or risk—personal or otherwise—that is incurred as a consequence, directly or indirectly, of the use and application of any of the contents of this book.

The Experiment's books are available at special discounts when purchased in bulk for premiums and sales promotions as well as for fund-raising or educational use. For details, contact us at info@ theexperimentpublishing.com.

Library of Congress Cataloging-in-Publication Data

Names: Fraser, Ruthie.
Title: Stack your bones : 100 simple lessons for realigning your body and
    moving with ease / Ruthie Fraser.
Description: New York : The Experiment, LLC, [2017]
Identifiers: LCCN 2016050274 | ISBN 9781615191987 (hardcover)
Subjects: LCSH: Posture. | Exercise--Physiological aspects. | Yoga.
Classification: LCC RA781.5 .F73 2017 | DDC 613.7/8--dc23
LC record available at https://lccn.loc.gov/2016050274

ISBN 978-1-61519-198-7
Ebook ISBN 978-1-61519-389-9

Cover and text design by Sarah Smith
Author photograph by Evan Sklar

Manufactured in China
Distributed by Workman Publishing Company, Inc.
Distributed simultaneously in Canada by Thomas Allen & Son Ltd.

First printing May 2017
10 9 8 7 6 5 4 3 2 1

Contents

PART 1: STRUCTURE

PART 2: BASIC MOVEMENT

PART 3: APPROACH

PART 4: CONTEMPLATIONS

Foreword
by Cyndi Lee

When I close my eyes and travel back in time to the days when Ruthie Fraser regularly attended classes at OM Yoga Center, my yoga studio in downtown Manhattan, I see a young woman with her own blend of composure, uprightness, and presence. Ruthie didn't come to class to get more stretchy, or buff, or to sweat out the stress of her work day. She came to study and practice.

In this wonderful new book, *Stack Your Bones*, Ruthie now transmits to us the joy and wisdom inherent in the various practices and modalities of which she is an expert. And many they are: She is a yogini trained in the methods of Iyengar, Ashtanga, Kripalu and OM yoga; dancer; certified yoga teacher; and Structural Integration practitioner.

Ruthie's experience of working and living into each of these paths—as a mover and a teacher, as a spiritual seeker, and as a movement guide—has led her to discover the most essential work for those of us who are not professional dancers or full time yogis, but simply have a body and *need* to move it.

These 100 "seeds," as Ruthie calls her lessons, integrate beneficial commonalities of various techniques and blend them with the same qualities I remember her bringing to her own work: clarity, intelligence, and confidence.

Clarity: In *Make It Simple* (lesson 56), Ruthie's message is clear and simple: "Eliminate extraneous complexity."

Intelligence: Ruthie points us to the innate wisdom of our own body and encourages us to bravely open to that which is good and right about us already. No need to push, pull, or improve, only to wake up and apply lessons on *Appropriateness* (lesson 61) and *Discernment* (lesson 62): learning to understand our needs—today.

Confidence: In *Order Under Disorder* (lesson 4), Ruthie gives a beautiful teaching that no matter how we are feeling at any given time, we can relax with things as they are: "You do not need to acquire anything—it's all there, underneath."

Drawing on the yogic practice of energetic duality, Ruthie also offers a series of paired teachings. My favorite pair is *Be Pieces* and *Be Whole*. What a gift to be reminded that sometimes we are in pieces, and that's part of our truth. And sometimes we naturally feel whole. Why not pay attention to that, too? Ruthie writes: "Contemplate your body as a vibrating, living whole."

I like these lessons. You can apply them to your own movement practice or you can work with them as you are waiting in line at the grocery store. *Stack Your Bones* not only helps us find our way back into our body—no matter when or where we are—but also shepherds us through the process in a way that allows us to feel comfortable in our own skin. This is a message that we all need to hear and receive. Ruthie understands that the only path to making friends with our body is to go through the body. She also knows that there is not just one way. In fact, in this book, she gives us 100.

CYNDI LEE is the first female Western yoga teacher to fully integrate yoga asana and Tibetan Buddhism in her practice and teaching. The founder of NYC's OM Yoga Center (1998–2012), she teaches worldwide and at her home studio, Yoga Goodness Studio, in Virginia. She is author of the yoga classic *Yoga Body Buddha Mind* and *May I Be Happy*, a memoir about body image and meditation, and also writes for *Yoga Journal*, *Real Simple*, *Lion's Roar*, and *Yoga International*. Cyndi is a long-time student of Gelek Rimpoche and a graduate of Upaya Buddhist Chaplaincy program under the auspices of Roshi Joan Halifax.

Introduction

Your body is intelligent. It knows how to beat your heart, breathe, digest food, regenerate cells, fight sickness, and perform innumerable other biological miracles. And it knows how to move, too. Your body is designed for comfortable movement. It's equipped and wired for natural, easeful alignment and coordination. However, as you move through life, your body's posture and movement functionality will sometimes veer off course. *Stack Your Bones* provides fun and simple ways for you to constructively influence your body's path.

Your body's shape and movement patterns continually change in response to the content of your life. These adaptations are not necessarily problematic; they are the natural ways your body compensates and evolves in the face of stress and challenging circumstances. Think of a tree that must reckon with a boulder that blocks its natural growth path: The tree will curve and wind itself around the boulder in order to survive in that context, demonstrating the instinctive resilience and creativity of living bodies.

But sometimes adaptations intensify or escalate, leading to excess strain, muscle dysfunction, and discomfort. Your body might spiral more out of alignment than your joints can tolerate. Or, an adaptation might persist beyond its original cause—for example, you might start limping because of an injury and then continue to limp even after your injury heals. Similarly, your body might tense up from emotional stress and "hold on" to this tension long after the upsetting situation has passed. Additionally, adaptations in your body may cause you to unintentionally perpetuate disadvantageous form or movement patterns during exercise.

I see adaptations in alignment and movement every day. I practice a system of bodywork called Structural Integration (SI), which aims to help a person regain flexibility, stability, efficiency, and resilience in their body. SI uses specialized manipulation of body tissues to evoke harmony in your body structure and freedom in movement, and capitalizes on your body's natural capacity to adapt positively.

While working with clients to help them overcome troubling patterns and thrive in their bodies, I created essential "lessons" rooted in Structural Integration principles. I gradually identified and developed the lessons that most stimulated experiential learning and contributed to comprehensive body wellness. Over the course of days, weeks, months, and years in my Structural Integration studio, a methodology formed. I am thrilled to share the foundations of the *Stack Your Bones* methodology with you in this book.

The 100 lessons of *Stack Your Bones* are not just exercises or stretches; they teach foundational principles that will help you understand your body and establish healthy patterns. Think of them as 100 seeds that you can plant in your body and your consciousness. Each lesson is brief but can have a big impact. These lessons will help you:

- cultivate and maintain comfortable, healthy body alignment and posture

- improve your muscle coordination and overall movement patterns

- gain a foundational understanding of body structure

- improve your body awareness and proprioception

- study and understand your body's imbalances and constitutional tendencies

- heal and transform muscular and postural patterns in your body that cause discomfort

- engage in a movement practice that is nourishing and speaks to your unique needs

- develop constructive playfulness and improvisation skills in movement

- evolve and elevate your definition of fitness

- apply useful teachings to your favorite physical activities

- feel fulfilled and enriched by the process of exploring and improving your body

I encourage you to search for personal meaning in each lesson. Ask yourself, "What might this lesson mean for me and my body? How do I relate to this teaching?" It's a playful and challenging journey to embark on. Make friends with your body! Acknowledge and appreciate all that your body has been through, as well as its intrinsic beauty. So, ignite your curiosity, commit to full participation, and have a good time! Who knows what will sprout from the soil?

Ruthie Fraser

December 2016

Ways to Use This Book

There are many valid ways to use the *Stack Your Bones* lessons in your life. Here are a few suggestions, and I invite you to come up with your own.

1. **Sequential practice.** Practice each lesson starting from number 1. Try one or several at a time in the order in which they appear. Though every lesson stands alone, the book offers a logical sequence.

2. **Daily practice.** Open the book randomly to any lesson. Let this lesson be a project for your day.

3. **Applied practice.** The lessons are compatible with any movement form. Choose a lesson, or a few lessons, and apply them in your favorite physical activity.

4. **Paired practice.** There are several pairs of lessons that balance and complement each other philosophically and physically. Practice the

pairs listed here, or find any two lessons that make an intriguing practice set. Suggested lesson pairs in order of appearance: *Mobility* and *Stability* (pages 40 and 42); *Differentiation* and *Integration* (pages 50 and 52); *Constructive Flexion* and *Constructive Extension* (pages 134 and 146); *Wild Body* and *Refined Body* (pages 204 and 206); *Be Pieces* and *Be Whole* (pages 208 and 210).

5. **Balanced practice.** Choose an equivalent number of lessons, from each of the four parts: *Structure*, *Basic Movement*, *Approach*, and *Contemplations*. Practice this sequence.

6. **Focused practice.** Choose several lessons from the same part for a sequence that focuses on *Structure*, *Basic Movement*, *Approach*, or *Contemplations*.

7. **Group practice.** Create a practice circle with some friends. Take turns opening the book to a random lesson, or plan a sequence of lessons based on your interests.

8. **For bodywork and movement professionals:** Incorporate *Stack Your Bones* lessons into your work. This book is a great tool for yoga teachers, Pilates teachers, fitness trainers, and body-oriented therapists.

PART 1

Structure

Experience the basic structure of your body
as a human and as an individual.

1
Stack Your Bones

Organize your body.

In a standing position, feel your skeleton. Don't worry about exact anatomy.

Stand with your feet directly under your sitz bones. Bring your shin bones directly under your thigh bones. Bring your pelvis directly over the arches of your feet.

Relax your buttocks, belly, back, and shoulders. Slowly and gently stack your spine from bottom to top. Bring your head directly over your tailbone.

Breathe. Do less. Let your body relax with gravity.
See what happens next.

"Form and function are a unity, two sides of one coin. In order to enhance function, appropriate form must exist or be created."
—Dr. Ida Rolf

2
Gravity
as an Asset

With well-stacked bones, it's good to be weight-bearing.

In a standing position, feel the weight of your body. Does the weight of your body feel good anywhere? Does it feel grounded or solid? Does it feel uncomfortable anywhere? Heavy or compressed?

Gently adjust to improve your body's architecture. Bring your feet and legs under your trunk. Bring your pelvis directly over the arches of your feet. Let go of excess muscle effort. Stack your bones and relax.

Can you feel the force of gravity as an asset? If you lived in outer space, there would be no uprightness.

"We want to get [you] into the place where gravity reinforces [you] and is a friend, a nourishing force."—Dr. Ida Rolf

3
Natural Human Posture

Good posture is effortless.

Stand with your legs and feet under you for support.

For a few moments, practice what you've learned about posture. Maybe you learned to lift your chest or pull in your belly. Maybe you learned to press your shoulders down or tuck your pelvis.

Now undo all of this, and try something else. Gently organize your bones. Relax. Get grounded. Soften the muscles around your pelvis and shoulders. Energetically feel the length of your body.

Does uprightness emerge? It will become more effortless as you cultivate body balance.

"Another aspect of erect posture is that it is a biological quality of the human frame and there should be no sensation of any doing, holding, or effort whatsoever." —**Moshe Feldenkrais**

4
Order Under Disorder

Your body has an underlying order.

Visualize your body's underlying order—your innate blueprint for healthy alignment and comfortable movement.

Do you feel layers of tension or dysfunction covering up that order? Imagine shedding layers you don't need. Relax and let go.

You do not need to acquire anything—it's all there, underneath.

"I saw the angel in the marble and carved until I set him free."
—Michelangelo

5
The Line

Orient to the vertical axis
that runs through your center.

Stand with your legs and feet under you for support.

Visualize a vertical line that runs through your center. The line travels down toward the center of the earth and up toward the sky and beyond.

Feel your body's organization or disorganization around The Line. Can you create more balance?

Don't overwork. Be gentle.

"Forget anatomy and take on art and you'll look at a body as a something around a line, a vertical line."—**Dr. Ida Rolf**

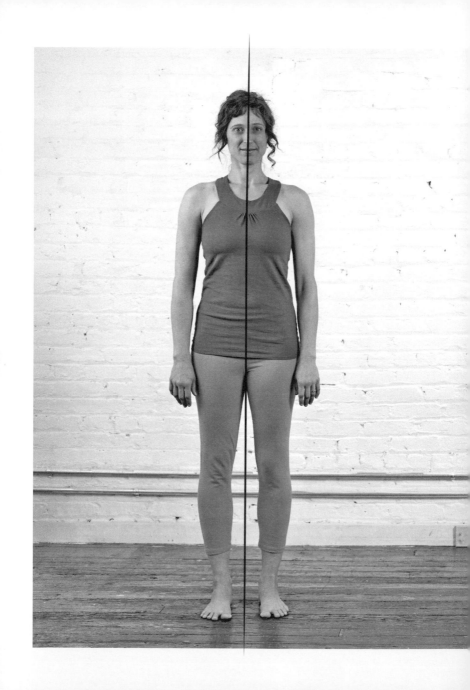

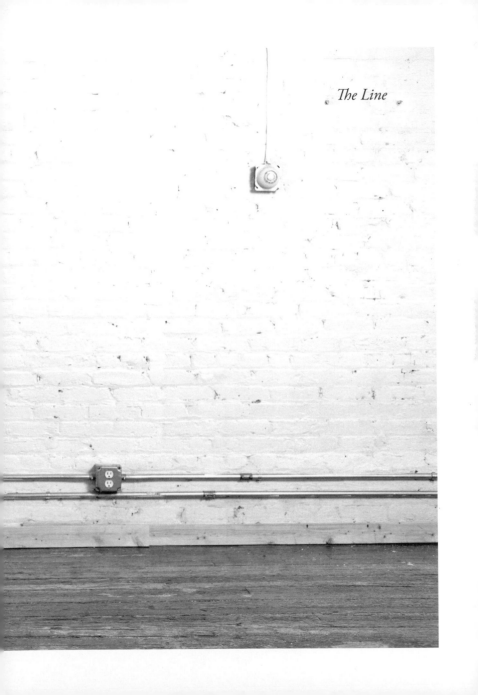

The Line

6
3D Grid

Relate to horizontal and vertical lines to get your bearings.

Stand with your legs and feet under you for support.

Feel your height from feet to head. This is the x-axis. Orient your spine in the x-axis.

Feel your width from side to side. This is the y-axis. Orient your collar bones and elbows in the y-axis.

Feel your depth from back to front. This is the z-axis. Orient the gaze of your eyes, your navel, and your kneecaps in the z-axis.

Relate to each axis in the grid. Feel your height, width, and depth.

"There is a mystical virtue in right angles. There is an unspoken morality in seeking the level and the plumb."
—Scott Russell Sanders

7

Aggregate of Segments

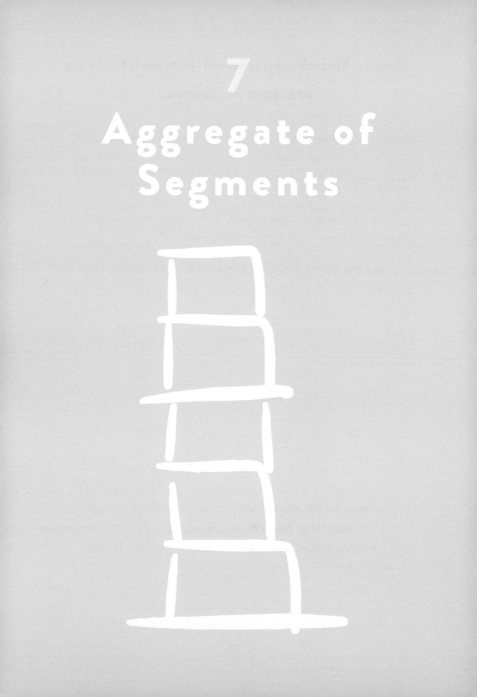

Your body is a collection of stacked segments.

Feel the stacked segments of your body. Feel your feet, shins, thigh bones, pelvis, abdomen and lower back region, rib cage, neck, and head.

Do any segments feel too far forward? Too far back? Right or left? Twisted, shifted, or tilted? If one segment goes forward, another is likely to go backward. If one shifts to the right, another is likely to shift to the left.

Body segments need support from underneath. It's easier to rest with a reliable foundation.

Play with gentle adjustments to restore natural relationships in your body.

"Depending on the structure of the body on which it acts, gravity can either support us and provide a springboard for our activities or it can pull at us and tear us down."—**Joseph Heller**

8
Span

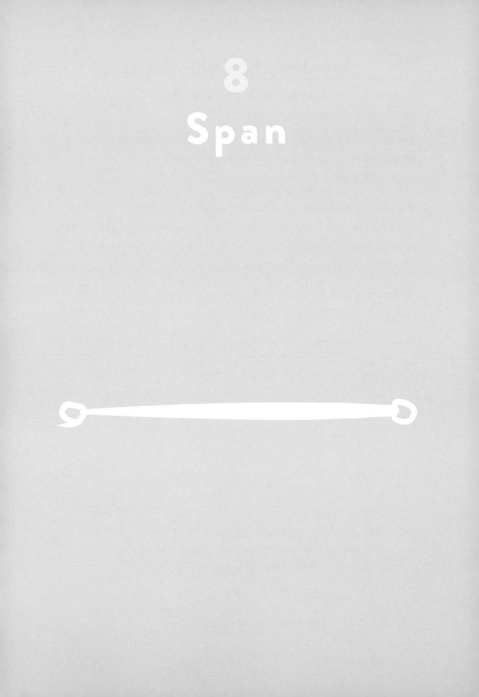

A balanced body has good spatial relationships.

Stand with your legs and feet under you for support.
Bring your attention to the inner landscape of your body.

Feel the distance between your pelvis and your rib cage.
Is there enough space there? Feel the distance between your
pubic bones and your sternum. Is there enough length there?
Is there too much?

Contemplate the spatial relationships in your body by scanning
distances.

"Your stability relies in appropriate relationships, and that is all."
—Dr. Ida Rolf

9
Fascia

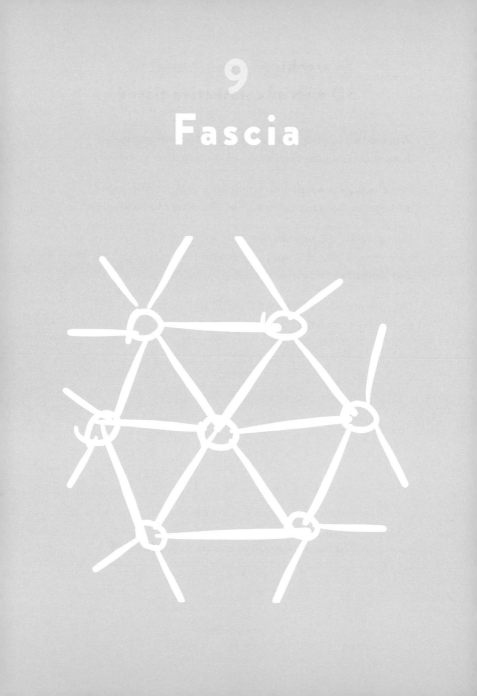

Everything is contained in a 3D web of connective tissue.

Visualize all of your body parts as contained in a multi-dimensional web of fascia.

If the web gets warped, shortened, or twisted, the bones, muscles, and organs contained in that web will be affected.

Take a walk. Feel your bones, muscles, and organs as structures contained within the web. If the web is balanced, the muscles and bones will float in natural alignment.

Do your muscles and bones float? Do they feel pulled or shifted by the web?

"Fascia is the organ of posture."—Dr. Ida Rolf

10
Tensegrity

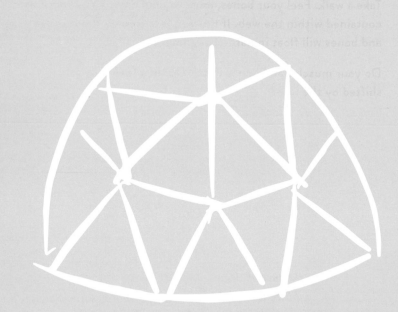

Cultivate equivalent tensional force around each joint.

Stand with your legs and feet under you for support. Feel your shoulder area.

Shrug your shoulders up toward your ears. Then press your shoulders down. Now bring your shoulders forward. Then bring your shoulders back behind you. Repeat. Notice the different muscles responsible for each of these actions.

Balanced muscle tone around joints creates equivalent tensional force in all directions.

Do your shoulders float inside balanced tensional force? Is there more tug in one direction than another?

"Support is a balance of elements that aren't solid at all, elements that are incapable of withstanding the weight that presses down on them except as they are balanced."—Dr. Ida Rolf

11
One Net

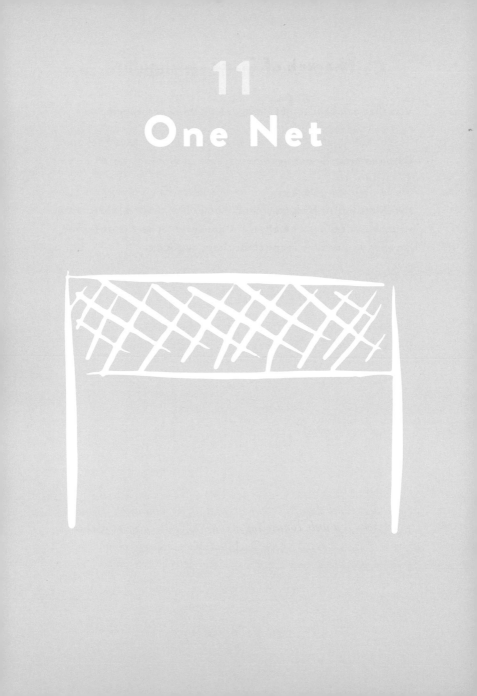

The web of fascia is singular.

Visualize a volleyball net. Imagine pinching and tugging one part of the net.

Observe how the net becomes warped and pulled, even on the opposite side.

Experience your body as a three-dimensional net with multiple surfaces, containing all of your body parts. Where might you have an original pinch and a consequential pull?

"A body is a web, connecting everything with everything else."
—Dr. Ida Rolf

12
Chain Reactions

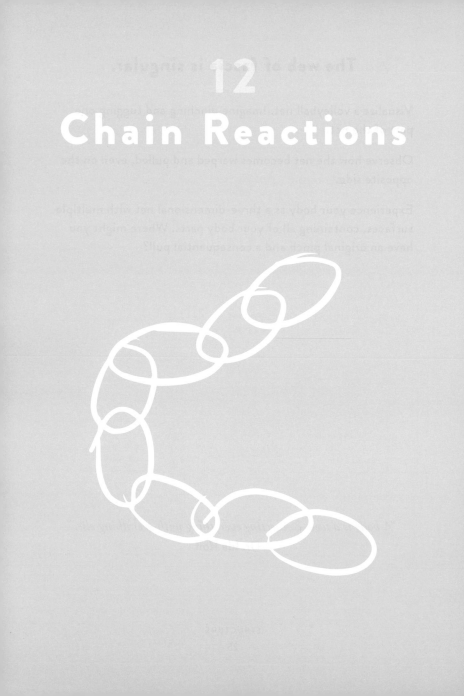

Aberrations cause more aberrations.

Stand with your legs and feet under you for support.
Bring your attention to the inner landscape of your body.

For a few moments, grip your buttocks and tuck your pelvis.
Does this cause tension or misalignment in other parts of
your body?

Now stick out your buttocks way too much. Does this cause
tension or misalignment in other parts of your body? Feel how
one aberration can lead to dysfunction in other places.

Can you apply the teaching of begetting aberrations to any of
your discomforts? Can you trace a pain or injury back along
the chain?

The good news is that chain reactions happen in healing too.

"One thing goes awry, and its effects go on and on and on and on."
—Dr. Ida Rolf

13
Chicken
and Egg

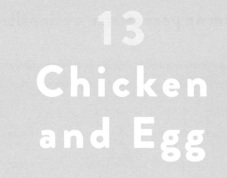

Patterns perpetuate each other.

If your pelvis is held in a tuck, it shortens your abdominal muscles. If your abdominal muscles are shortened, it pulls your pelvis into a tuck.

Who knows which came first? The patterns are linked.

Here's another example: If your pelvis is tilted anteriorly, it shortens your lower back. If your lower back is shortened, it tilts your pelvis anteriorly.

Do you have any chicken-egg patterns in your structure?

"The body process is not linear, it is circular; always, it is circular."
—Dr. Ida Rolf

14

Division
of Labor

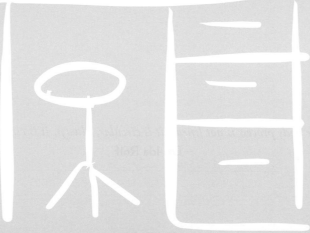

Each body part has a job.

Overworked muscles get tired and cranky. They compensate for lazy or inhibited muscles. Sometimes they compensate for unstable areas in the skeleton.

Which muscles overwork in your body? Which don't work enough?

Contemplate an environment in which each muscle does its proper job—no more, no less.

The same is true for joints. If one joint becomes stuck, another one will become too loose to compensate.

15
Cooperation

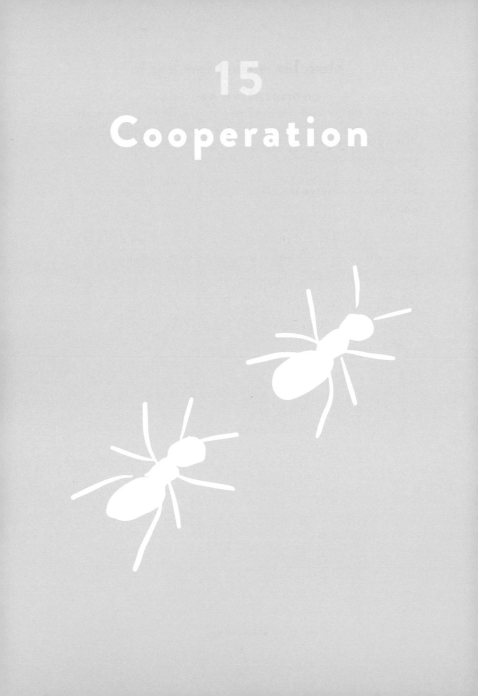

Muscles work together in cooperative groups.

Bring your attention to the inner landscape of your body as you go for a walk.

Slow down. Observe the elemental movement components of walking.

Feel one knee lift and the foot reach forward. Feel the ball of your other foot press into the ground. Feel your weight shift. Feel the subtle swing of your arms.

Contemplate the individual muscles responsible for each action and the cooperation required to move naturally.

16
Lively Muscles

Relaxed, healthy muscles perk up.

Find a comfortable position. Bring your attention to your face.

For a few minutes, give yourself a face massage. Apply gentle pressure to your forehead, temples, cheekbones, and jaw. Press into the flesh of your face and make circles with your fingertips.

How does your face feel now?

Relaxing muscles through touch, stretching, or awareness is rejuvenating and enlivening!

17
Availability

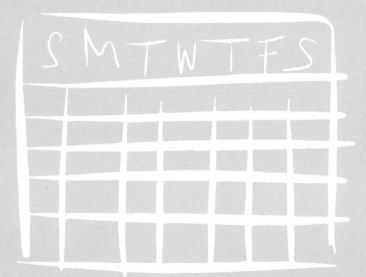

Relaxed, aligned muscles are available for use.

Find a comfortable position. Bring your attention to the inner landscape of your body.

Are any muscles in your body contracted or misplaced? Do your buttocks clench all the time? Are your shoulders pulled forward?

When a muscle grips unnecessarily or exists in the wrong place, its strength is inaccessible.

Focus on unclenching and restoring alignment to make all muscles available.

18
Strength Is Balance

Balanced strength is real strength.

Come to your hands and knees. Lengthen your spine. Extend your elbows. Bring your knees directly under your hips and your hands directly under your shoulders.

Round your entire spine. Tuck your pelvis and tuck your chin. This is spinal flexion, created by spinal flexors.

Next, arch your spine to create a backbend. Lift your buttocks, elongate your abdomen, and lift your chest and chin. This is spinal extension, created by spinal extensors.

Is one direction easier for you?

When flexors and extensors throughout the body (and all opposing muscle groups) are balanced in strength, then the body is resilient.

"A prerequisite for chronic pain is a habitual imbalance of muscle usage around a particular joint or joints. Some of the muscles crossing a joint are weaker than others, some are stronger. There is a situation of relative weakness but not of absolute weakness."
—Irene Dowd

19
Mobility

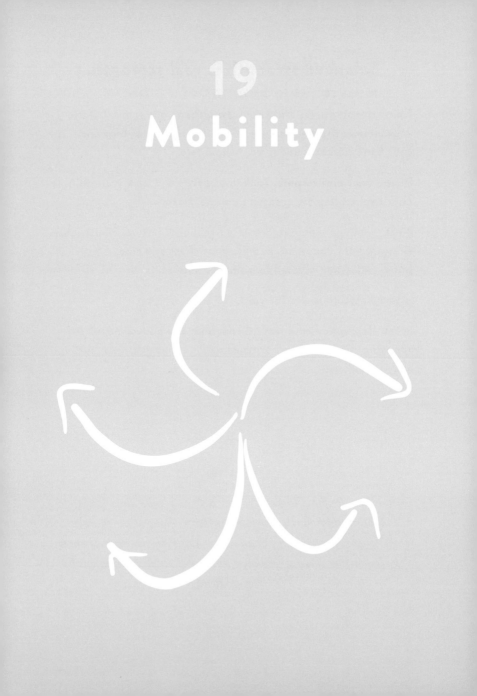

A resilient structure possesses a reasonable amount of mobility— throughout.

Flex and extend your elbows. Notice how the movement of the joint has a range of motion.

If your elbow could not bend or straighten at all, it would be stuck.

Contemplate the need for mobility in order for the body to be functional.

20
Stability

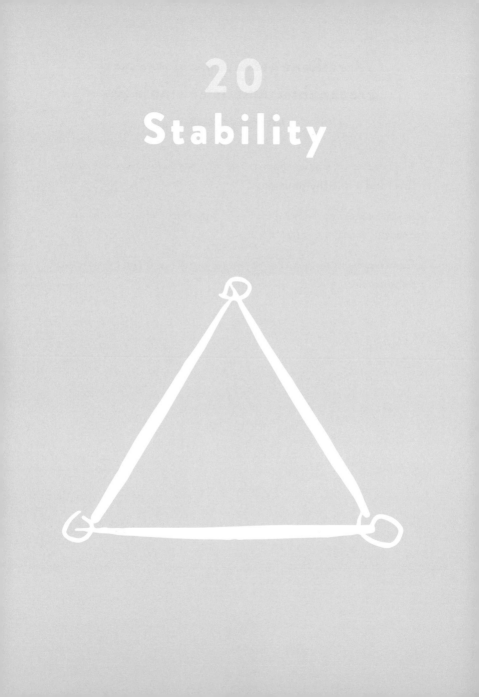

A resilient structure possesses a reasonable amount of stability—throughout.

Flex and extend your elbows. Notice how the movement has a limit and a healthy pathway.

If your elbow could swing in infinite directions, it would be unstable.

Contemplate the need for limits on mobility in order for the body to be functional.

21
Layers

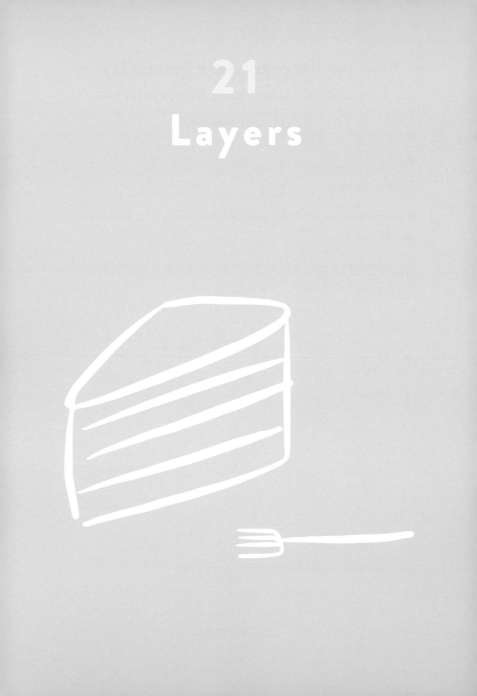

Your body is composed of many layers.

Bring your attention to the inner landscape of your body as you prepare for an experiment.

Put on a formfitting T-shirt. Twist your T-shirt in random ways.

Put on another T-shirt over the first one; twist this one in different ways. And put on another.

Do the same with three layers of legging or pants.

The body's layers can get twisted up. Learn to unwind layer by layer.

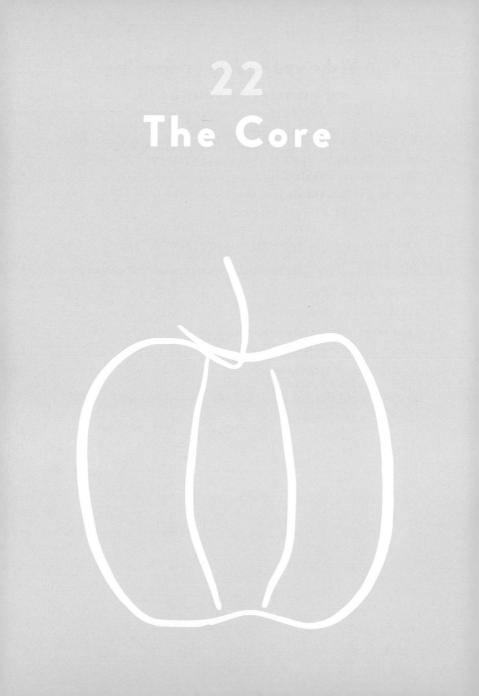

22
The Core

Wake up the deepest family of muscles in your body.

Lie down on your back. Bend your knees, and place your feet on the floor as far apart as your hips. Adjust your flesh so that your whole back feels long. Rest your palms on the floor near your hips. Allow the floor to support your body.

Imagine a central tube in your body, similar to the cylindrical core of an apple. Bring your awareness into this "apple core" of your body.

Core muscles inhabit and potentially animate your central tube. Visualize your deepest spinal muscles. Tune in to your psoas muscles and deep abdominal muscles. Feel the muscles of your pelvic floor. Feel your diaphragm and internal intercostal muscles as you breathe slowly.

Are your core muscles awake? Do they engage automatically? Can you activate them on command?

23
Core and Sleeve

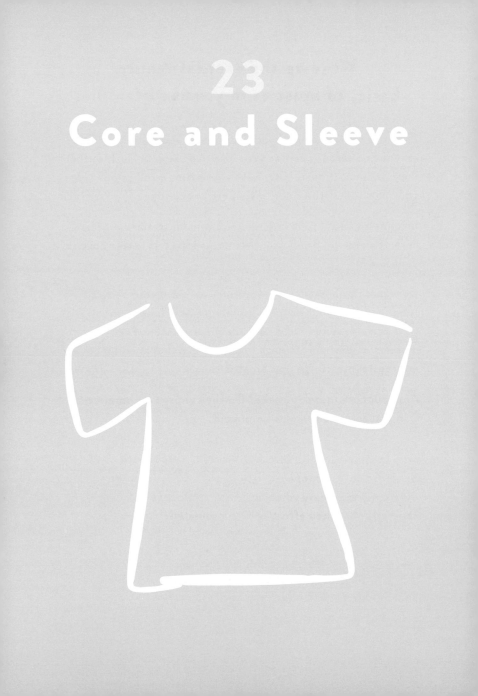

Activate and coordinate two basic, complementary muscle families in your body.

Lie down on your back on the floor. Adjust your flesh so that your whole back feels long. Spread your arms and legs into a big X.

Feel your arms and legs, as well as the shell of your trunk—the outer layers of your back, buttocks, abdomen, and chest. This is your *sleeve*.

Now bend your knees and place your feet on the floor as far apart as your hips. Rest your palms on the floor near your hips. Allow the floor to support your body.

Feel the "apple core" of your body—your deep spinal muscles, your deep abdominal muscles, your psoas muscles, your diaphragm, your internal intercostal muscles, and your pelvic floor. Visualize an awake, active core.

As a healthy pair, the core and the sleeve are functionally distinct and also cooperate in movement. Do you utilize both your core and sleeve when you move? Are they balanced in strength? Are they effortlessly coordinated?

24
Differentiation

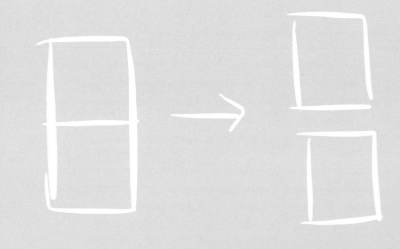

Cooperation first requires unsticking.

Bring your attention to the inner landscape of your body as you perform a simple physical task.

For example, reach for a plate. Are any muscles contracting that you don't need? As you lift your arm, do your buttocks unconsciously clench? Are you working too hard for such a simple exercise?

Reach for the plate using only the muscle effort you need for that action and no more.

Unstick extraneous actions from essential actions.

25
Integration

The parts of a structure can coordinate in harmony.

Bring your attention to the inner landscape of your body as you perform a simple physical task.

For example, open a door. Feel how this action involves your whole body. Notice your weight shift from foot to foot as you reach for the knob. Feel your trunk lengthen as you lift one arm. Feel the coordination of your legs, abdomen, and shoulders as you swing the door open and step through.

Contemplate your whole-body coordination. Could it be more efficient? More comfortable? More natural? More harmonious?

PART 2

Basic Movement

Explore the building blocks of healthy alignment and movement through elemental physical practices.

26
Constructive Rest

Rest in an organized, well-supported body.

Lie down on your back. Bend your knees, and place your feet on the floor as far apart as your hips.

Adjust your flesh so that your whole back feels long. Rest your hands on your belly or place your palms on the floor near your hips.

Feel how the floor can support your body.

Let go of tension. Surrender to gravity.

"All action begins in rest."—Lao Tzu

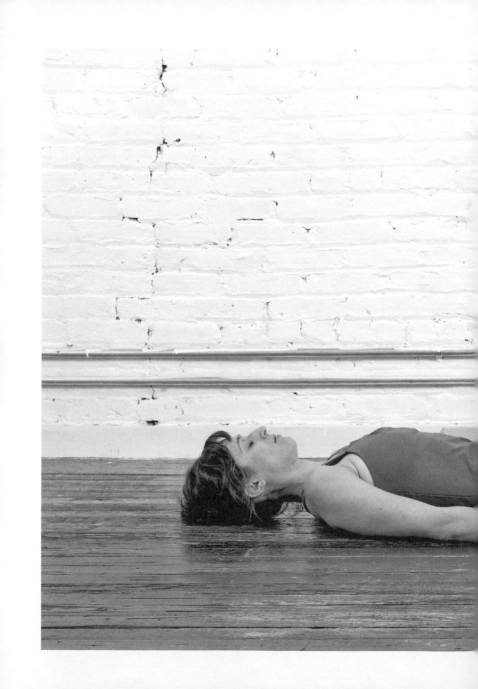

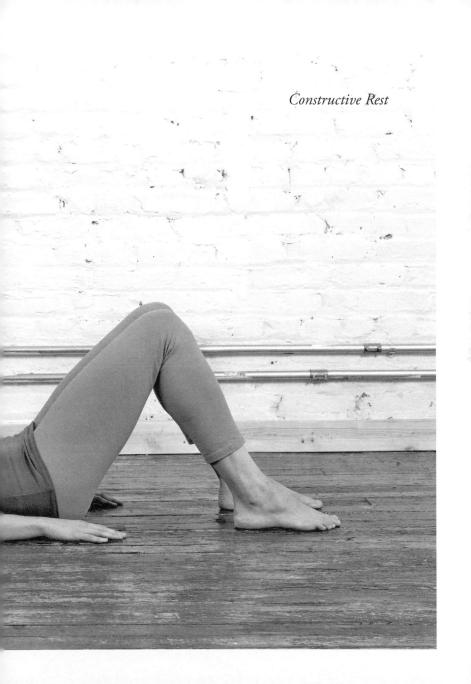

Constructive Rest

27
Find Your Feet

Drop into your feet for essential support.

Lie down on your back. Bend your knees, and place your feet on the floor as far apart as your hips. Adjust your flesh so that your whole back feels long. Rest your palms on the floor near your hips. Allow the floor to support your body.

For a moment, lift your feet an inch off the floor. Feel how several muscles in your body contract in order to maintain the position.

Place your feet down again. Consciously use your feet on the floor in order to let go in the rest of your body.

Grounded feet make relaxation possible.

28
Tuck and Arch

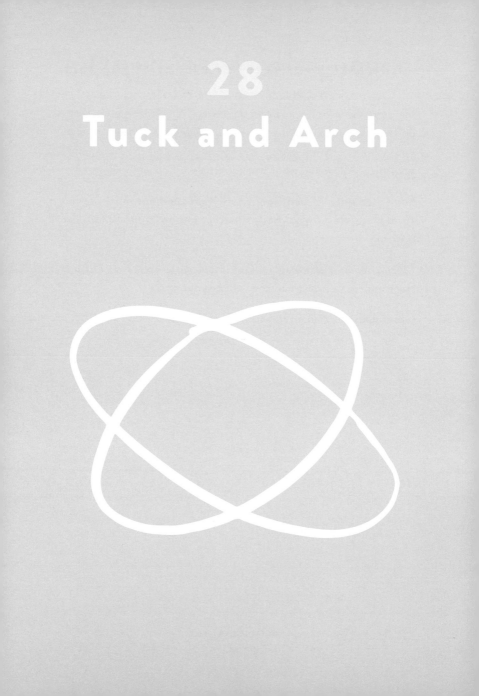

Master the movement of your pelvis in two basic directions.

Lie down on your back. Bend your knees, and place your feet on the floor as far apart as your hips. Adjust your flesh so that your whole back feels long. Rest your palms on the floor near your hips. Allow the floor to support your body.

Tilt your pelvis so that your tailbone points up and the top of your sacrum presses down into the floor. You will also feel your lower back press into the floor. This is a *tuck*.

Now tilt your pelvis so that your tailbone points down and the top of your sacrum lifts away from the floor. You will also feel your lower back lift away from the floor. This is an *arch*.

Tuck and arch again. Move slowly and smoothly back and forth, passing through a neutral, balanced pelvis in between. Try to use the support of your feet and minimal muscle effort.

29

Pelvic Floor Diamond

Get to know the bony borders of your pelvic floor.

Lie down on your back. Bend your knees, and place your feet on the floor as far apart as your hips. Adjust your flesh so that your whole back feels long. Rest your palms on the floor near your hips. Allow the floor to support your body.

Find your pubic bones with your fingertips. Then slide your hand under your buttocks and find the tip of your tailbone with your fingertips. Next, find the bottom of the right sitz bone and the bottom of the left sitz bone.

These are the four corners of your pelvic floor. Focus on the space inside the diamond, which includes layers of musculature, your genitals, and your anus. This is your pelvic floor.

Make small movements with your pelvis, following the bony landmarks in your mind.

30

Pelvic Clock

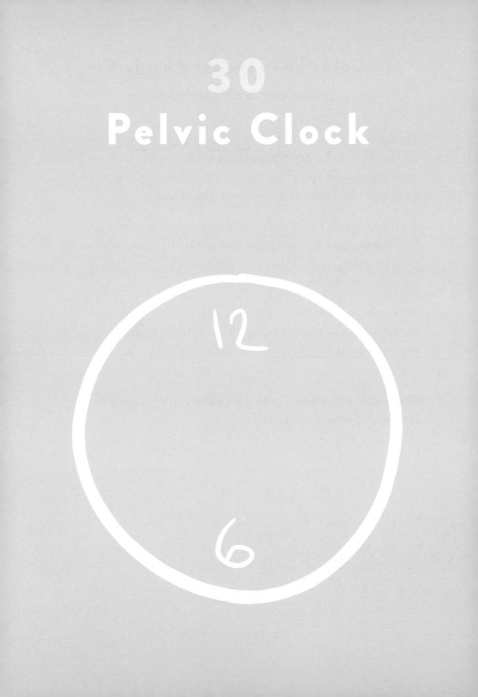

Move your pelvis in specific directions for agility and precision.

Lie down on your back. Bend your knees, and place your feet on the floor as far apart as your hips. Adjust your flesh so that your whole back feels long. Rest your palms on the floor near your hips. Allow the floor to support your body.

Imagine a marble in the center of your pelvis. Roll the marble in the direction of your tailbone. Feel how your pelvis tilts into an arch. This is twelve o'clock.

Roll the marble in the direction of your abdomen. Feel how your pelvis tilts into a tuck. This is six o'clock. Roll to twelve o'clock and then to six o'clock, passing through the center of the clock.

Roll the marble to various numbers. Try one o'clock to seven o'clock, passing through the center. Try eleven o'clock to five o'clock. Continue and create your own patterns. Improvise.

31
Balanced Pelvis

A balanced, neutral pelvis floats.

Stand with your legs and feet under you for support.

Play with the position of your pelvis relative to surrounding body parts (thigh bones, abdomen, lower back). Tilt your pelvis anteriorly into an arch. Tilt it posteriorly into a tuck.

Move your pelvis in various directions. Feel the range of motion of the pelvis.

Are certain directions easier for you than others? Notice the tendency of your pelvis.

Explore a centered position for your pelvis. Can your pelvis float in neutrality?

"The combined forces acting on a balanced pelvis are in a moment of inertia near zero. It is always in dynamic action, but the forces balance out to near zero." —Dr. Ida Rolf

32
Eight Grounding Points

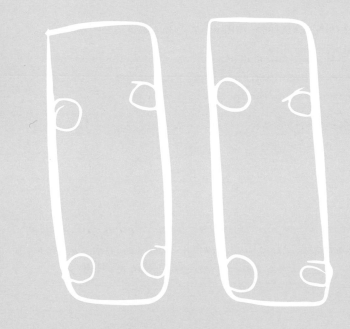

Evenly distribute your weight among the four corners of each foot.

Stand with your legs and feet under you for support. Bring your attention to your feet. Where does weight drop through your feet?

Lift and spread your toes.

For each foot, feel the inner ball of the foot (at the base of the big toe). Feel the outer ball of the foot (at the base of the little toe). Feel the inner heels and outer heels.

Now relax your toes, and feel the four corners of each foot.

For a moment bring all of your weight into the two inner corners of each foot. Then bring your weight into the two outer corners of each foot. Notice your tendencies.

Balance your weight on the four corners of each foot. Be in your whole body.

33
Inner Heels,
Inner Legs

Root your inner heels;
wake up your inner legs.

Stand with your legs and feet under you for support.

Imagine each of your heels as a circle on the floor. Divide each circle in half, into inner and outer halves. Imagine the inner half of each circle grounding down toward the center of the earth.

Notice how this compares to how you usually stand.

From your grounded inner heels, draw lines of energy up your inner legs to the pelvic floor.

Activate your inner legs. Let your inner legs support your trunk.

34
Legs as Columns

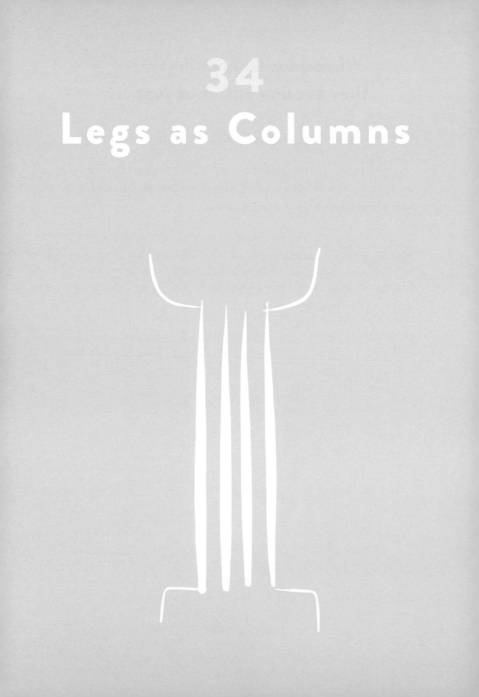

When your legs are organized, they become pillars of support.

Come to a standing position. Bring your attention to your legs.

Bring your feet directly under your sitz bones. Bring your shin bones directly under your thigh bones.

Unwind and organize your feet, ankles, shins, knees, and thighs without causing strain.

Create column-like, supportive legs.

With this supportive architecture in place, you can eliminate extraneous muscle gripping throughout your body.

35

The Bell

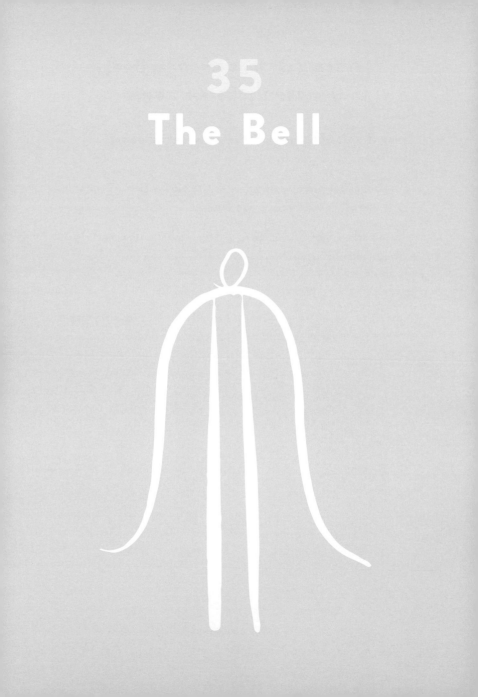

Your legs fall from your diaphragm like the clapper of a bell.

Stand with your legs and feet under you for support. Bring your attention to your feet.

Move your awareness up your legs and thighs. Don't stop at your hips. Travel the awareness of your "legs" all the way to your rib cage.

Feel your diaphragm, a dome-like muscle at the base of your rib cage. Allow these extra-long legs to descend from your diaphragm.

Allow your legs to undulate to and from your diaphragm as you move.

36
Adjacent
Cylinders

Bring length and awareness to the right and left halves of your body.

Stand with your legs and feet under you for support.

Lift your arms overhead. Vigorously extend your arms and legs while lengthening your trunk.

Imagine the right half of your body as a continuous cylinder from the right foot up through the right leg, the right side of the trunk, and the right arm. Imagine the same on the left.

Feel your body as two adjacent cylinders.

Feel the interior space of each cylinder. Imagine a vertical midline running through each cylinder. Elongate, energize, and organize the midlines. Experience them as long, bright, and parallel.

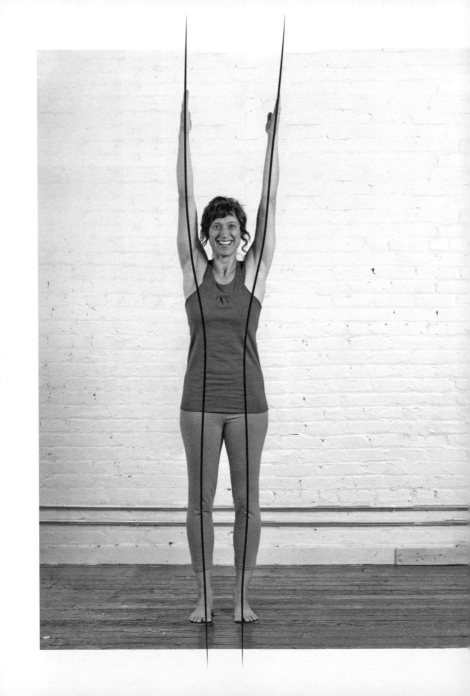

Adjacent Cylinders

37
Root and Expand

Get grounded for ascension and expansion.

Stand with your legs and feet under you for support.

Root your feet and legs.

Let your body surrender to gravity. Notice if an effortless lift emerges, rising up through your body and expanding in many directions.

Play with the energies of rooting, surrendering to gravity, rising from within, and expanding multidirectionally.

"If we surrendered to earth's intelligence we could rise up rooted, like trees."—Rainer Maria Rilke

38
Domes of Lift

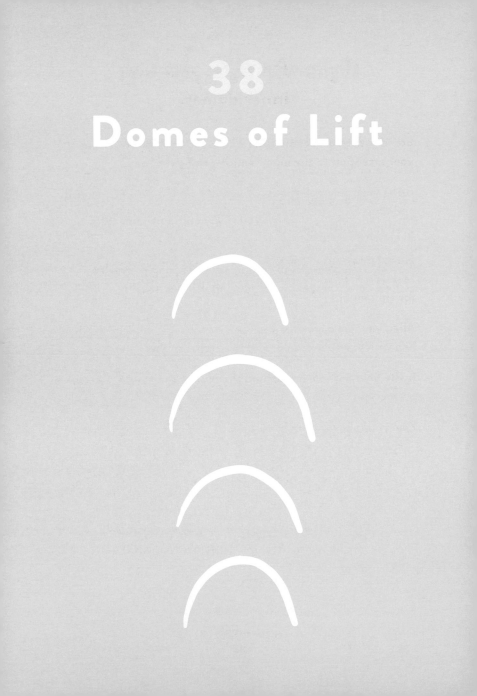

Align and energize your body's inner domes.

Stand with your legs and feet under you for support. Bring your attention to the inner landscape of your body.

Bring your pelvis all the way forward over the balls of the feet and toes. Observe. Next, bring your pelvis all the way back over your heels. Observe.

Now, bring your pelvic floor directly over the arches of your feet. Activate your arches by lifting and spreading your toes for a moment.

Align your rib cage over your pelvis to bring your diaphragm in line with your pelvic floor and the arches of your feet.

Invite your soft palate, behind the roof of the mouth, to stack on top.

Feel your domes of lift perk up.

39

Buoyant
Shoulders

Let your shoulders float.

Stand with your legs and feet under you for support.
Bring your attention to your shoulders.

Let go of any "doing" or "fixing" in your shoulders.

Shrug your shoulders up toward your ears. Feel how this
elongates your side ribs. While shrugging, wiggle your
shoulders in many directions.

Now relax your shoulders without pushing them down.
Gently lift your side ribs up toward your underarms.

Create a subtle buoyancy in your shoulders, inspired by
the space and freedom of the shrug and supported by your
ascending side ribs.

40
Centered
Shoulders

For balanced shoulders, float the heads of your upper-arm bones evenly in their sockets.

Stand with your legs and feet under you for support. Bring your attention to your shoulders.

Let go of any "doing" or "fixing" in your shoulders.

Shrug your shoulders up toward your ears. Now direct your shoulders down as much as you can. Next, bring your shoulders all the way forward. And then bring them all the way backward.

Repeat these movements, feeling into the different parts of your shoulder sockets. Play with the full range of motion of your shoulders.

Now explore a neutral place where your shoulders are not shrugging up, pushing down, moving forward, or going backward.

Where do your shoulders feel centered?

41
Wide Elbows

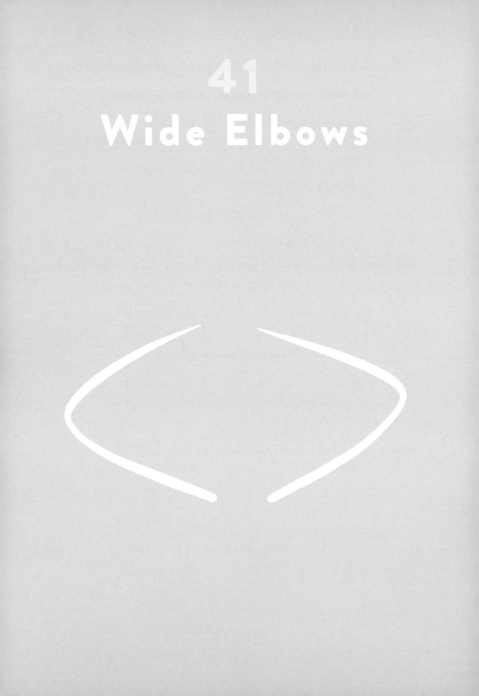

To organize your upper body, orient your elbows to the sides.

Stand with your legs and feet under you for support. Bring your attention to your shoulders.

Let go of any "doing" or "fixing" in your shoulders.

Place your hands on your hips, orienting your elbows to the sides. Gently elongate your spine. Allow your elbows to widen as extensions of your back.

Now let your arms hang down. Continue to orient your elbows to the sides. Face your inner elbows in and your outer elbows out. Let the palms face back. Relax and center your shoulders.

Breathe into any resistance. This position might feel strange or challenging at first. As you practice wide elbows, you can unwind the arms, shoulders, and neck.

"Our arms start from the back because they were once wings."
—Martha Graham

42
Hanging Arms

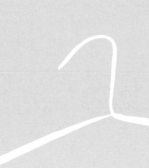

Let your arms hang loosely.

Stand with your legs and feet under you for support. Feel your shoulders, neck, and arms.

What are your arms doing? Do they hang loosely or are they held up in tension?

Extend your arms to your sides at shoulder height. Widen your wingspan, and feel the stretch. Then lift your arms to create a wide V above your shoulders. Stretch from the center of your back up through your arms.

Lengthen your spine as you continue to stretch your arms vigorously in the high V. Extend your elbows and fingers. Soften your shoulders.

Now relax your arms by your sides again. Do they hang looser after the stretch? Play with letting go in your arms.

43
Head on Top

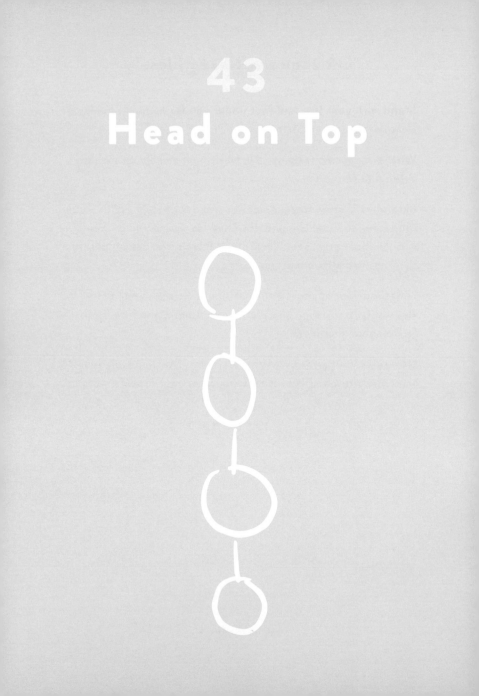

Bring your head in line.

Stand with your legs and feet under you for support. For a moment, bring your hands to your head.

With your hands, feel the shape of your head. Touch the back, sides, and top of your head.

Now let your arms hang down. Feel the location of your head relative to the rest of your body. Is it too far forward? Is it tilted?

Shift your attention down to your feet. Get grounded. Soften your body. Relax around your pelvis. Create a gentle lift through your spinal column. Gently adjust the position of your shoulders, chest, and neck.

Be in your whole body. Stack your head right on top.

44
Top Half of the Head

Stand in your full height.

Stand with your legs and feet under you for support. Bring your attention to your head.

Notice the placement of your eyeballs. Many of us stand as if we are only as tall as the height of our eyes.

Feel into the space of your head above your eyeballs. There's a lot more height there!

45
Tracking

Practice elemental movements with healthy alignment.

In a standing position, bring your attention to your pelvis and legs.

Organize your feet, ankles, shins, knees, and thigh bones under your pelvis.

Slowly bend your knees slightly. Notice where they are headed. Are your knees tracking straight over your feet? Are they parallel?

You may feel your knees' tendency to go off center. You may feel resistance in your ankles or hips.

Reset and try again. Bend your knees a little bit, tracking them straight forward over each respective foot. Simultaneously reach your sitz bones straight back—just a little. As much as your knees lengthen forward, lengthen your sitz bones back.

Track your knees back to straight legs. Repeat the exercise. Move slowly and smoothly.

"When your car's wheels are misaligned, driving and turning them more will not improve matters; in fact, until you realign them, further movement will only increase the damage being done to your vehicle."—**Joseph Heller**

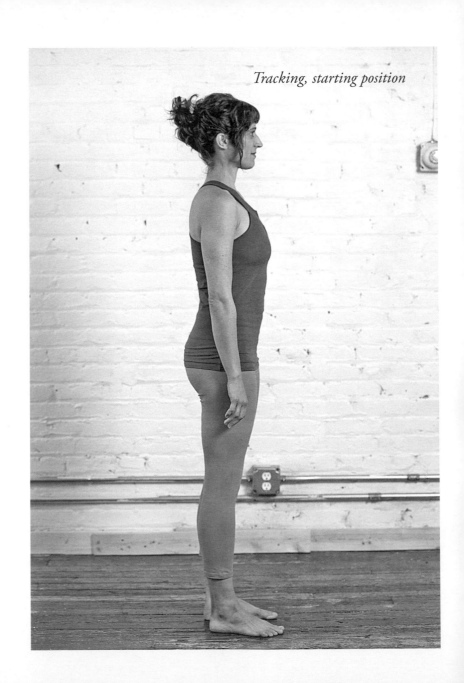

Tracking, starting position

Tracking

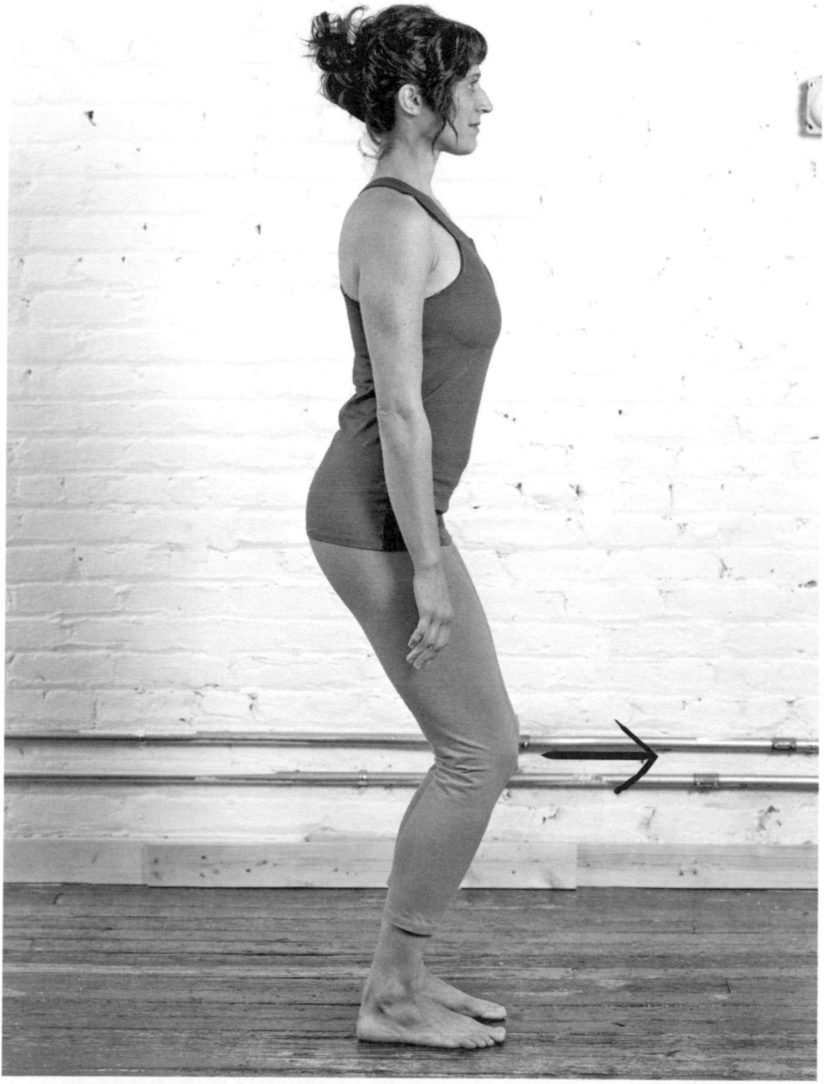

46
Sit Well

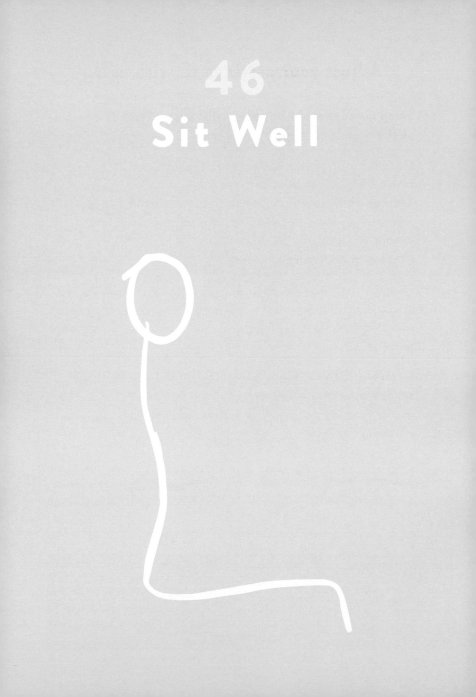

Adjust your pelvis to sit with ease.

Sit on the edge of a chair with parallel thighs. Place your feet on the floor directly under your knees.

Move the flesh of your buttocks back behind your sitz bones. Take some time to play with the position of your pelvis. Do not tuck your pelvis at all. Instead, tilt the front of your pelvis down slightly and make sure your buttocks are behind you. If your pelvis tilts easily, be careful not to overdo it. Sit directly on the center of your sitz bones.

Elongate your abdomen and stack your rib cage over your pelvis. Gently lift your side ribs toward your underarms and let your shoulders float. Gently guide your head to stack over your spinal column.

Be present with any resistance or tightness in your body. Do not hold yourself up with muscle effort. Feel the floor under your feet and feel the chair under your sitz bones. Organize your body and relax.

47
Seated Hinge

Master a basic, elegant movement on your sitz bones.

Sit on the edge of a chair with parallel thighs. Place your feet on the floor directly under your knees.

Move the flesh of your buttocks back behind your sitz bones. Sit directly on the center of your sitz bones.

Elongate your abdomen and stack your rib cage evenly over your pelvis. Gently guide your head to stack over your spinal column.

Maintaining a stable spine, slowly hinge forward by creasing at your hips. Guide your trunk to stay long as it tips over your grounded sitz bones. Gently lengthen your sitz bones back as you hinge forward. Allow your thigh bones, led by your knees, to lengthen forward as you hinge forward. Return to center.

Hinge forward again and then return, practicing all of the components described above. Rotate your pelvis over your thigh bones to make a clean hinge.

"The paradox is that when a balanced body bends there is flexing movement but the body lengthens. There is no shortening."
—Dr. Ida Rolf

48
Head to Tail

Enliven the head-tail connection.

Come to your hands and knees. Lengthen your spine. Extend your elbows. Bring your knees directly under your hips and your hands directly under your shoulders.

Feel your head, and move it slowly. Let your head guide your neck, shoulders, and rib cage.

Feel your tailbone, and move it slowly. Let your tailbone guide your pelvis and lower spine.

Allow your head and tail to communicate in movement and mirror each other. Let your whole body respond and play.

49
Tail Wiggle

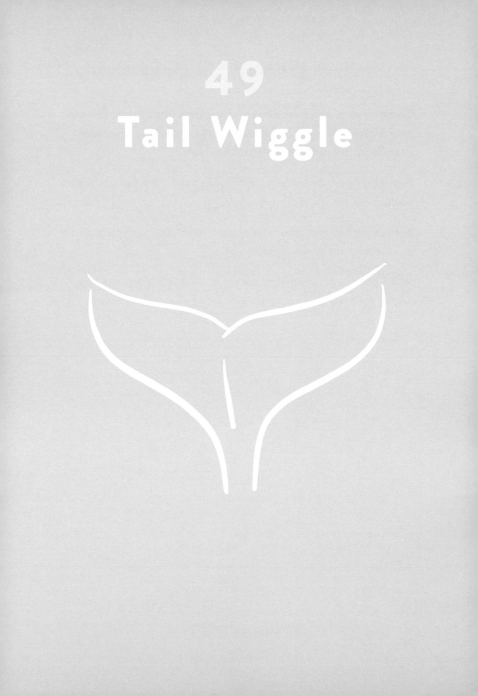

Move fluidly through the tip of your tail.

Come to your hands and knees. Lengthen your spine. Extend your elbows. Bring your knees directly under your hips and your hands directly under your shoulders.

Gently move your spine. Create wave patterns. Undulate.

Move the wave motion down toward your lower spine, sacrum, tailbone, and tip of your tailbone.

Initiate spontaneous movement with the tip of your tail. Let that movement reverberate back up your spinal column.

Feel the length of your spine when it includes your whole tail.

50
Undulation

Undulate for spinal health.

Come to your hands and knees. Lengthen your spine.
Extend your elbows. Bring your knees directly under your hips
and your hands directly under your shoulders.

Gently begin a wave motion in your spine. Don't rush. Let an
undulation pattern emerge and develop. Be slow and subtle
at first.

Continue to explore undulating your whole spine as you
breathe deeply. Allow the undulation to move in many
directions. Let it slow down to stillness and then start again.

Let your mind surf the waves of your body.

"You are only as young as your spine is flexible."—Joseph Pilates

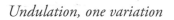

Undulation, one variation

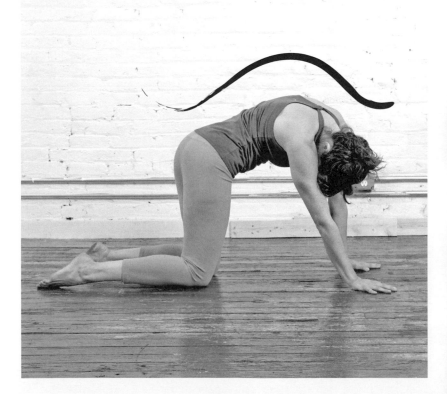

Undulation, another variation

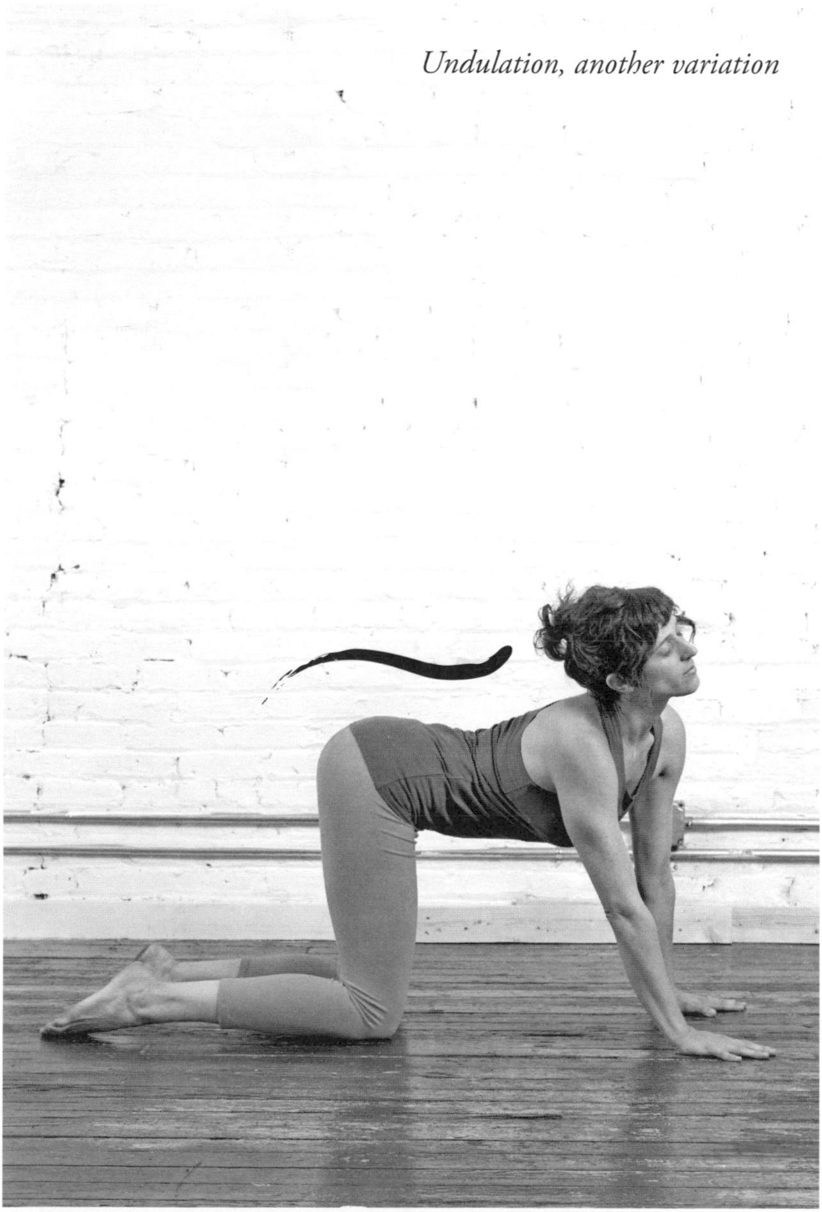

PART 3

Approach

Study the underlying values and strategies of a
constructive movement practice.

51

A Nourishing Orientation

Move your body for nourishment.

Attune yourself to a nourishing approach to movement and exercise.

What would feel nourishing for your body right now? A spontaneous variation of a yoga pose? A deep stretch? Stillness? A brisk walk?

Nourish your body with a kinesthetic activity of your choice.

52
Good Digestion

Nourishment requires fifty percent good food and fifty percent good digestion.

Lie down on your back. Bend your knees, and place your feet on the floor as far apart as your hips. Adjust your flesh so that your whole back feels long. Rest your palms on the floor near your hips. Allow the floor to support your body.

Extend your arms overhead along the floor. Open your hands and fingers. Lengthen your elbows. Extend your legs along the floor. Roll your thighs to orient your kneecaps straight up. Open your feet and toes. Lengthen your knees. Elongate your spine and abdomen. Breathe slowly and smoothly.

Can you internalize the instructions in your body? Can you digest them into nourishment?

"Experience teaches only the teachable."
—Aldous Huxley

53
Inner Awareness

Get to know what's happening.

Find a comfortable position. Be in the part of your mind that observes internally.

Observe the inner landscape of your body. Scan your whole body slowly. Remain open as you look, listen, and feel internally.

Make small, slow, gentle movements. Continue to observe.

Are you doing what you think you are doing?

*"If you don't know what you're doing,
you can't do what you want."*
—Moshe Feldenkrais

54
Close Attention

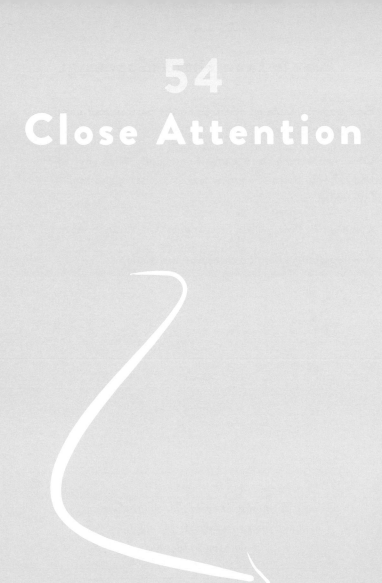

Tune in to details with curiosity.

Find a comfortable position. Bring your attention to the inner landscape of your body.

Bring your attention to a specific part of your body.

Light up that area with your attention. Observe the texture and sensations of that part.

Stay open to whatever thoughts, images, and feelings arise. Simply be present with whatever you find.

"The moment one gives close attention to anything, even a blade of grass, it becomes a mysterious, awesome, indescribably magnificent world in itself."
—Henry Miller

55
Do Less

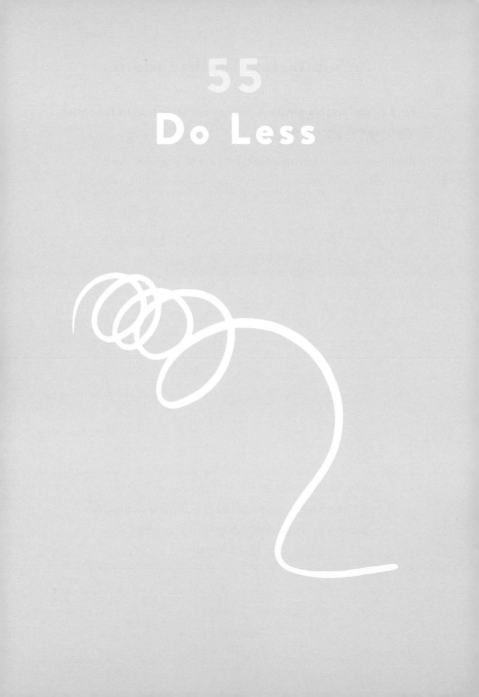

Subtract rather than add.

Find a comfortable position. Bring your attention to the inner landscape of your body.

Experiment with letting go of unnecessary tension and contraction. Where are you holding that you don't need to? Awareness can help you do less.

Play with this subtractive process. Observe.

In the absence of unnecessary doing, what's left?

"Everyone is always teaching one what to do,
leaving us still doing the things we shouldn't do."
—F. M. Alexander

56
Make It Simple

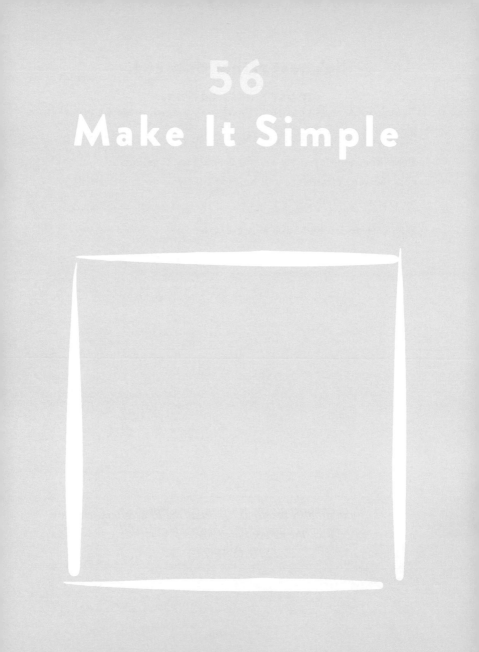

Reduce movements to their most basic forms.

In a standing position, bring your attention to your pelvis and legs.

Slowly bend your knees, tracking them straight forward over each foot. You may feel your knees' tendency to go off center or to zigzag around resistance in your body. Straighten your knees and pause.

Bend your knees again, and this time make it more simple. Move your knees straight forward and straight backward, without fuss. Eliminate extraneous complexity.

"The ability to simplify means to eliminate the unnecessary so that the necessary may speak."
—Hans Hofmann

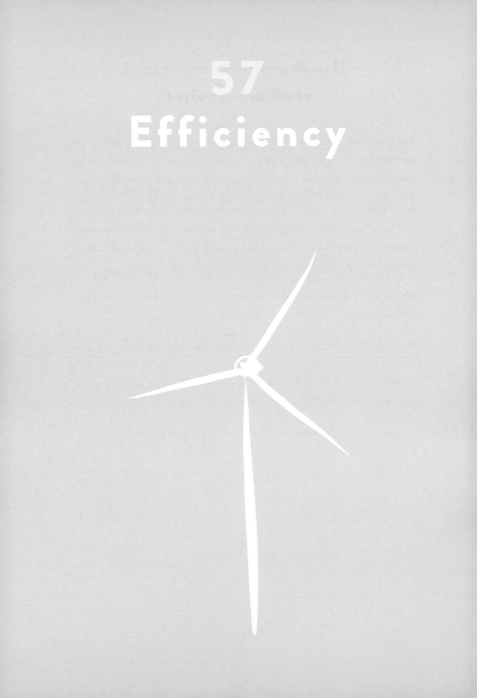

57

Efficiency

Use the minimum amount of effort required.

Lie down on your back. Bend your knees, and place your feet on the floor as far apart as your hips. Adjust your flesh so that your whole back feels long. Rest your palms on the floor near your hips. Allow the floor to support your body.

Tilt your pelvis so that your tailbone points up and the top of your sacrum presses down into the floor. You will also feel your lower back press into the floor. This is a *tuck*.

Move from a neutral position to a tuck and back to neutral. Observe.

Now repeat the tuck, but use minimal muscular effort. Do not harden your abdomen or buttocks. Let go of unnecessary gripping. Press your feet into the floor in order to tuck your pelvis. Be in your bones.

Utilize your well-aligned skeleton instead of extra muscles. Apply this to all movement. It saves energy!

58
Inner
Technology

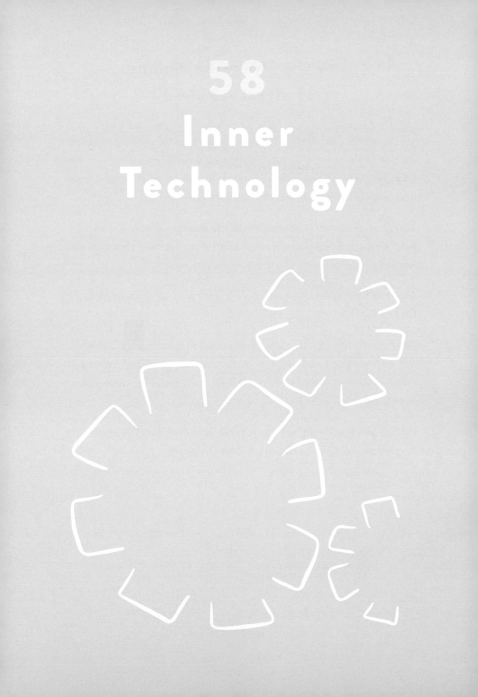

Revive your body's innate technology.

Stand with your legs and feet under you for support. Bring your attention to the inner landscape of your body, the floor, and the space around you.

Lift the arches of your feet to provide support for your whole body. Imagine a buoyant, supportive pelvic floor.

Take a walk. Contemplate the distinct job of each muscle. Feel the automatic coordination between various areas of your body.

Aim to restore your body's natural inner functionality. All the technology your body needs is within.

59
Vary Your Route

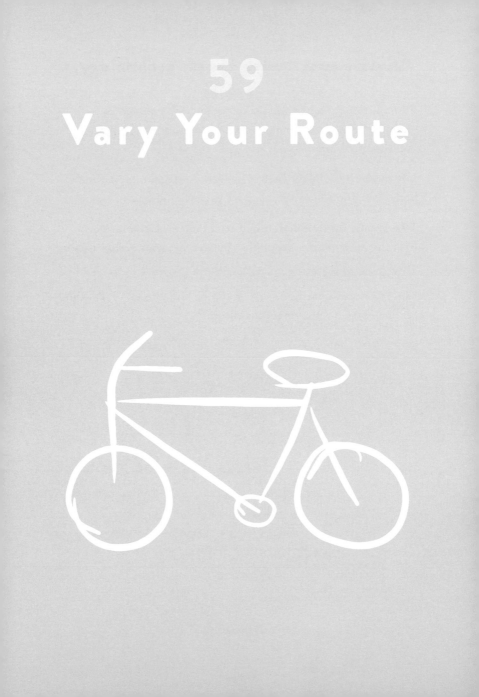

Diversify your movements to expand your capacity.

Come to your hands and knees. Lengthen your spine. Extend your elbows. Bring your knees directly under your hips and your hands directly under your shoulders.

For a few moments, move in a familiar way. Then, begin to improvise. Make a novel shape. Create a new pathway with your spine.

Follow an idea into a new universe of form and movement.

Habitual movements create habitual thinking. Feel your mind open as your body travels new routes.

"Venture from the known to the unknown."
—B. K. S. Iyengar

60
Constructive Flexion

Consciously round to open your back-body and soothe your nervous system.

Come to your hands and knees. Soften your abdomen. Breathe slowly.

Rest your buttocks back toward your heels to come into a "child's pose." Rest your forehead on the floor or a folded blanket. Rest your arms alongside your shins.

Let your back become very round. Let your shoulder blades separate. Create fullness in your back as your spine rounds.

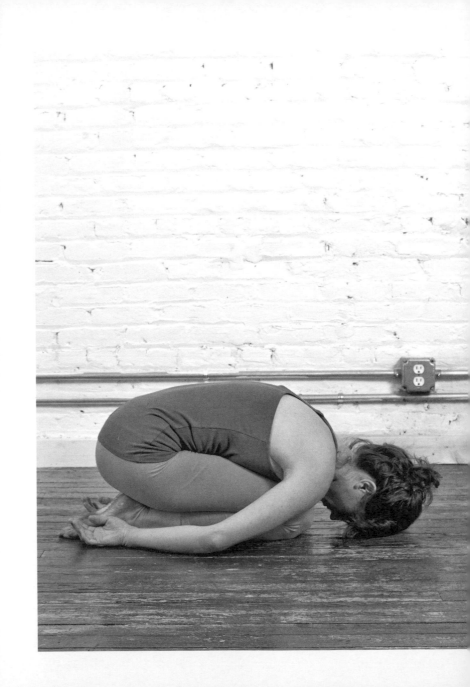

Constructive Flexion

61
Appropriateness

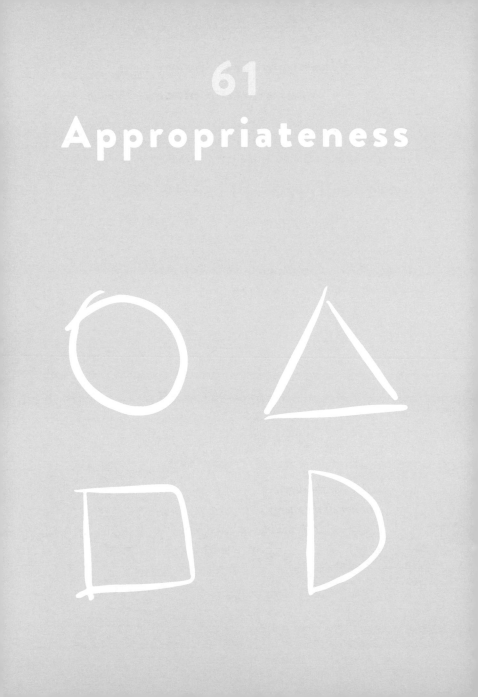

What you need depends on your starting place.

Stand with your legs and feet under you for support. Bring your attention to the inner landscape of your body.

If you're holding yourself up, let go and drop down.

If you're sinking, create a gentle lift from deep inside.

Before you exert yourself, contemplate what you are working toward. What's appropriate for your body right now?

"It is not the degree of 'willing' or 'trying,' but the way in which the energy is directed, that is going to make the 'willing' or 'trying' effective."
—F. M. Alexander

62

Discernment

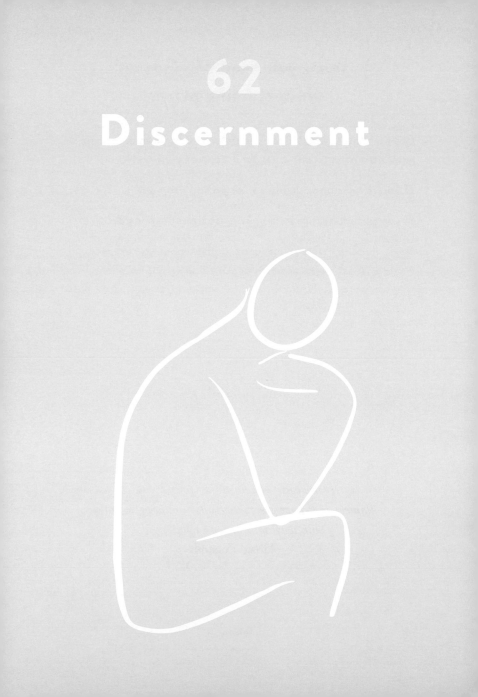

Evaluate what your body needs, here and now.

In a standing position, bring your attention to the inner landscape of your body.

Energize your body. Widen your eyes.

Pause and reflect. Are these cues appropriate for you? Were you already energized and wide-eyed? Would it be more useful for you to relax your body and soften your eyes?

Maybe the cues were appropriate, but only to a small degree. Learn to discern what's productive and relevant to you.

"There are two ways to slide easily through life:
Namely, to believe everything, or to doubt everything;
both ways save us from thinking."
—Alfred Korzybski

63

Tackle the
Imbalances

Strengthen what's weak and open what's tight.

Stand with your legs and feet under you for support.
Bring your attention to the inner landscape of your body.

Which areas of your body are the least flexible? Maybe your hamstrings or calves? Maybe your shoulders? If you aren't certain, it's worth exploring.

Spend more time stretching and opening those areas.
Move toward balanced flexibility.

Apply this to strength, too.

64
Un-Sink

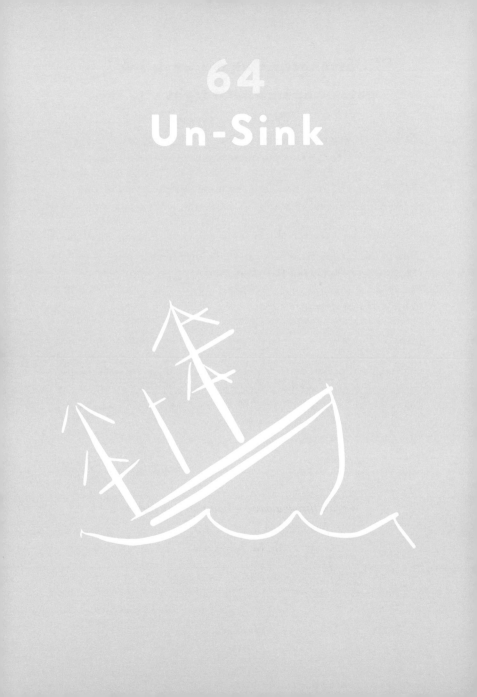

Without awareness you can sink into patterns; with awareness you can transform them.

Stand with your legs and feet under you for support.
Bring your attention to the inner landscape of your body.

Think of a pattern or tendency in your body. Maybe you
tend to stand more on the outer edges of your feet. Or on the
inner edges. Maybe you tend to tilt your pelvis anteriorly.
Or posteriorly. Maybe you tend to hunch your shoulders or
carry your head forward.

For a moment, exaggerate your pattern. Let yourself sink
into it.

Now, slowly pull yourself out of that pattern, and aim for more
balanced alignment. Be in your whole body. Be aware of the
floor under your feet.

Be gentle. Don't use too much muscle effort to un-sink.

*"We can throw away the habit of a lifetime in a
few minutes if we use our brains."*
—F. M. Alexander

65
Constructive
Extension

Consciously extend to energize and lengthen.

Find a bolster or create a stack of folded blankets. Lie on your back with the bolster or blankets under your rib cage.

Stretch the flesh of your back long as you lay on the support. Pull the flesh of your buttocks away from your rib cage to create traction. Reach your arms overhead toward the floor behind you.

Fully inhabit the supported backbend. Extend your fingers, toes, knees, and elbows. Make your limbs longer and brighter.

Elongate your trunk and extend your body. Breathe.

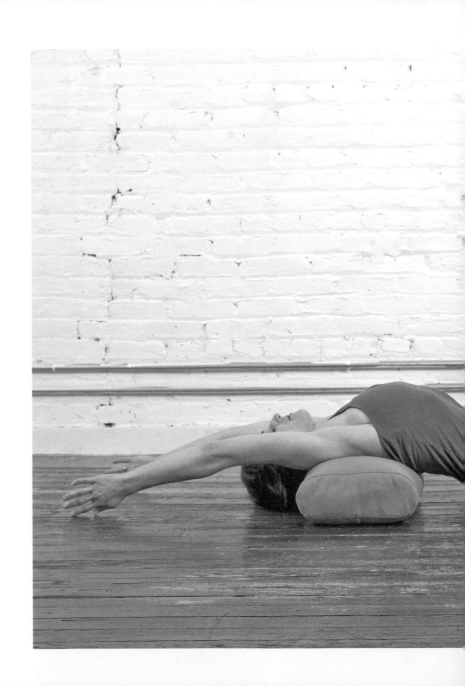

Constructive Extension

66
Floss Your Fascia

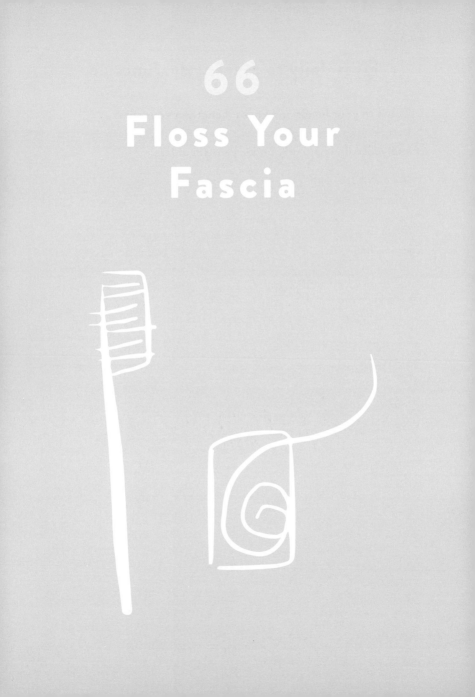

Floss daily to prevent dysfunction.

Come to your hands and knees. Lengthen your spine.
Extend your elbows. Bring your knees directly under your hips
and your hands directly under your shoulders.

Play with the full range of motion of your shoulders. Undulate
your spine. Make circles with your pelvis and your neck.

Move in a way that feels like flossing the plaque out of your
joints. Improvise.

When you feel some resistance, lean into it. Scrape it away
with your movements. Be gentle.

67
Think Globally

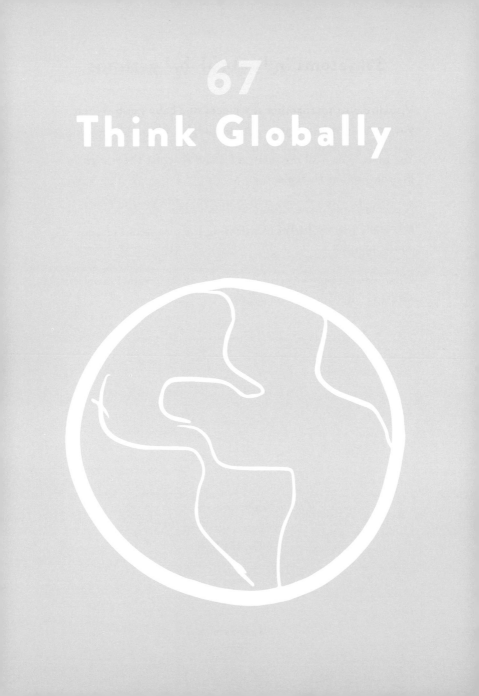

Symptoms indicate global patterns.

Visualize putting together the pieces of a baby's crib. When you come to the final joint, the pieces don't line up!

You must loosen all the joints a bit and readjust them slightly in order for the final pieces to align.

A problem might seem local, but it's usually global. How does this apply to your body?

"If it's somewhere in the body, it's everywhere in the body."
—Dr. Ida Rolf

68

Targeted Practice

Target a symptom by balancing your whole structure.

Visualize a tablecloth spread on a table. Picture a wrinkle in the middle of the cloth.

Imagine yourself smoothing out that wrinkle. What's your method?

You can pull on the ends of the cloth to eliminate the wrinkle. The whole tablecloth needs to shift just a bit to smooth out the wrinkle.

You don't need to touch the wrinkle directly to get rid of it. How might this relate to patterns in your body?

"Go around the problem; get the system sufficiently resilient so that it is able to change, and it will change."
—Dr. Ida Rolf

69

Investment

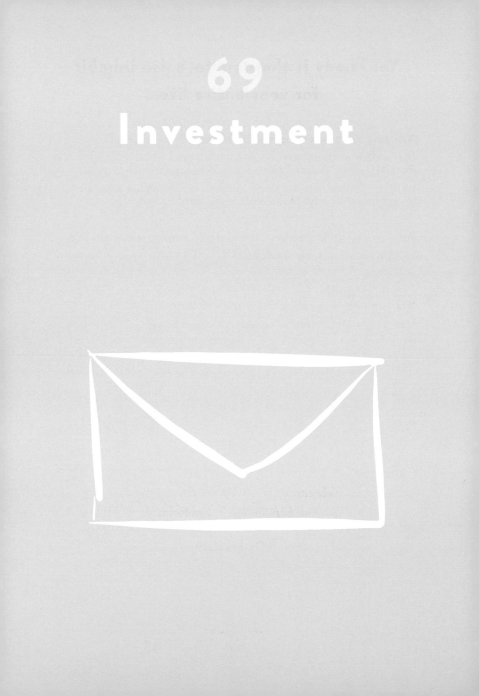

Your body is the structure you inhabit for your entire life.

Ask your body what it needs to thrive.

Rest? Healing? Touch? Movement? Therapeutics?

Invest in your body. Make a plan you want to follow.

"Take care of your body. It's the only place you have to live."—Jim Rohn

70
Cross-Training

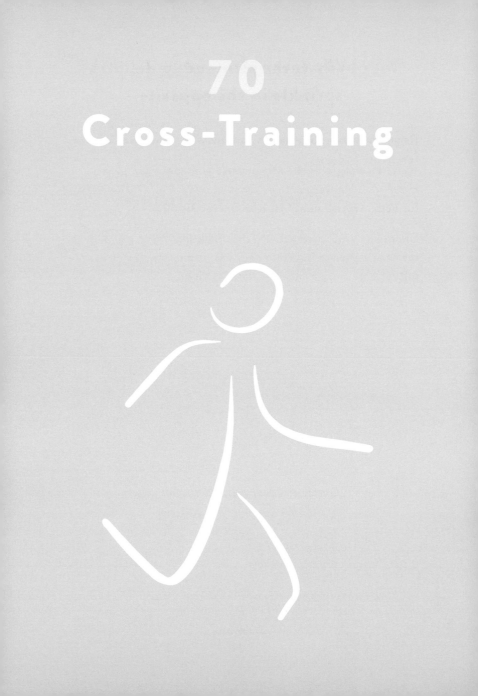

Whatever you tend to do, sprinkle in the opposite.

Recall how your body has spent most of its time in the past few hours or days.

Have you been very active? Or sedentary? Have you exercised for body nourishment? Have you stretched?

Choose an embodied activity that feels like cross-training for what's been going on in your life. It might mean deep relaxation; it might mean something vigorous. Enjoy.

71
Fine-Tuning

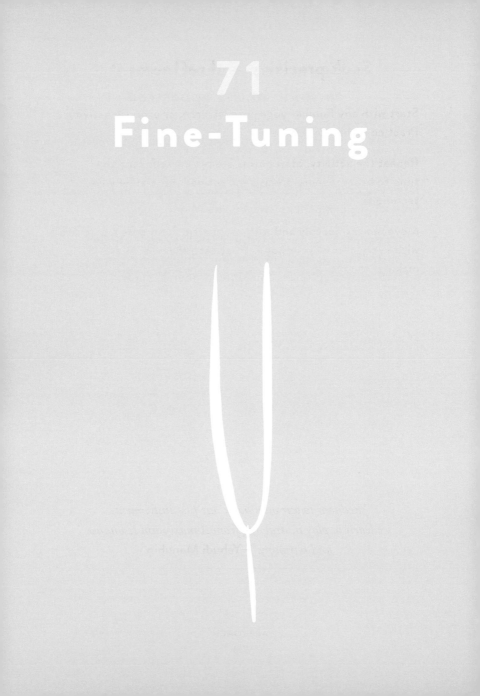

Seek precision and refinement.

Start with any familiar yoga pose, stretch, or exercise activity. Practice it the way you've learned.

Repeat the activity. Slow down. Study yourself. Take the time to become more precise and refined. Fine-tune your technique.

Move more smoothly and with more articulation. Be deliberate with every part of your body. Treat each moment as art-making.

"Reduced to our own body, our first instrument, we learn to play it, drawing from it maximum resonance and harmony."—Yehudi Menuhin

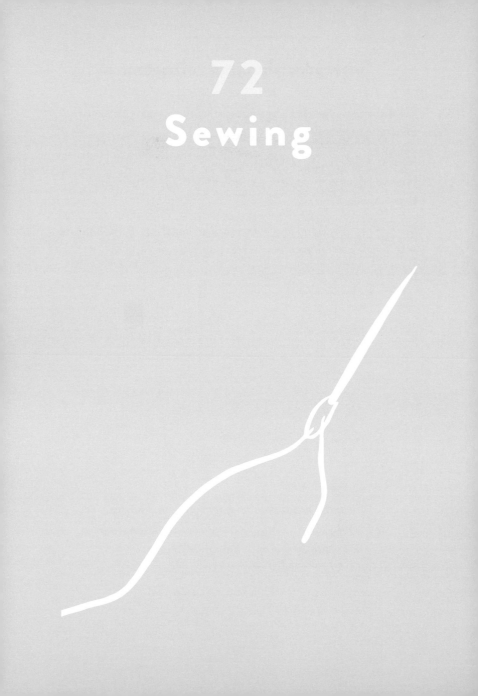

72
Sewing

Thread your actions together.

Lie down on your back. Bend your knees, and place your feet on the floor as far apart as your hips. Adjust your flesh so that your whole back feels long. Rest your palms on the floor near your hips. Allow the floor to support your body.

Extend your arms overhead along the floor. Open your hands and fingers. Lengthen your elbows. Extend your legs along the floor. Roll your thighs to orient your kneecaps straight up. Open your feet and toes. Lengthen your knees. Elongate your spine and abdomen. Breathe slowly and smoothly.

Repeat, threading all of these actions together. Sew one to the next, creating a continuous fabric of conscious action.

73
Skillful Play

Spontaneously respond to the moment.

Lie down on your back. Adjust your flesh so that your whole back feels long. Bring your attention to the inner landscape of your body.

Stretch out your arms, legs, abdomen, and spine. Breathe slowly.

Improvise. What does your body want to do? What's useful? Nourishing? Intriguing?

Dig deeper than habits and training.

"Lose your mind and come to your senses."
—Fritz Perls

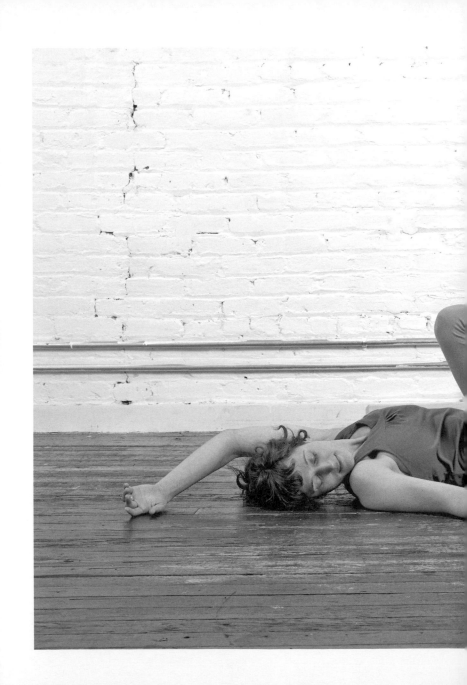

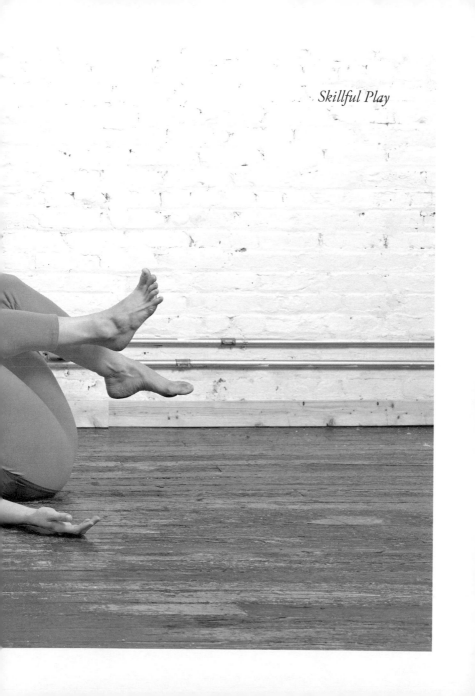

Skillful Play

74

Springboard

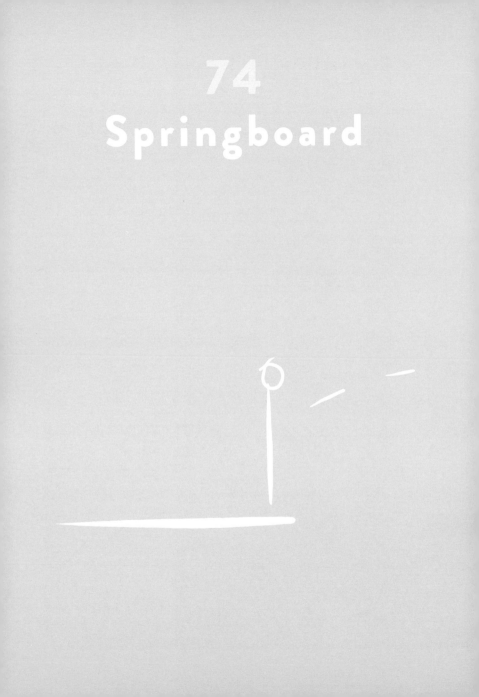

Every activity is a jumping-off point.

Start with any familiar yoga pose, stretch, or exercise activity. Practice it the way you've learned.

This is a starting place. Now dive into the experience.

Make it more personal. Invent a variation. Play.

Make it more relevant to you and more nourishing for your body in this moment.

"Imagination is the highest form of research."
—Albert Einstein

75
Body as Guide

Let your body guide you.

Pause. Take a break from telling your body what to do.

Listen. What does your body's voice say? What does it request?

For a few minutes, let your body be in charge.

"The body says what words cannot."—Martha Graham

PART 4

Contemplations

Inquire into the realms of emotion, kinesthetic qualities, and human nature.

76
Your Story

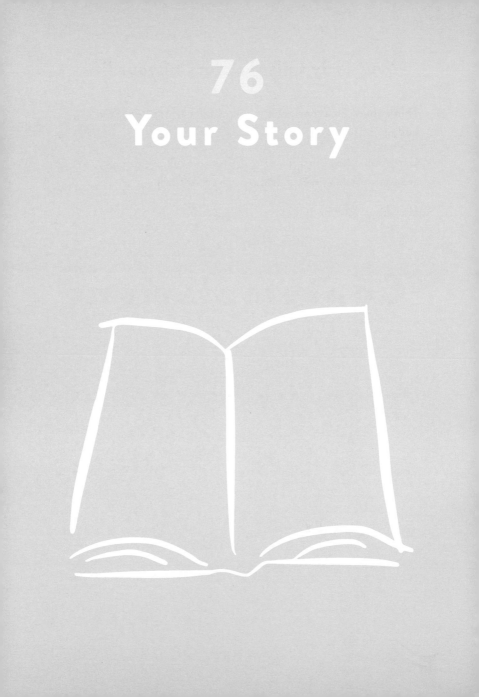

Your body tells the story of your life.

Think about an experience in your life that has impacted your body.

Can you feel the residue of this experience in your body? What are the sensations there? Stay with it for a while.

How does your body express this experience?

77
Rings of a Tree

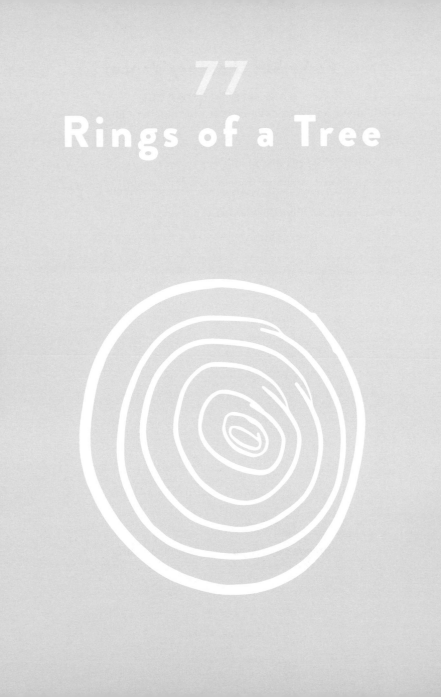

Your body holds evidence
of a life sequence.

What has your body experienced in the past year? Explore how your body tells your story.

Now think about the previous year. What happened then? Does your body indicate those experiences?

Go back further. Feel how your body records your story through time, like the rings of a tree.

"We meet ourselves time and again in a thousand disguises on the path of life."—Carl Jung

78

Bottled-Up
Emotions

Your body is charged with emotion.

Think about a time when you experienced a particularly strong emotion. For a few moments, enter that emotional universe.

Where do you feel the emotion in your body? What are the sensations there?

Breathe into the sensations and the emotion. Watch them change, move, or shift. Stay with them for a while.

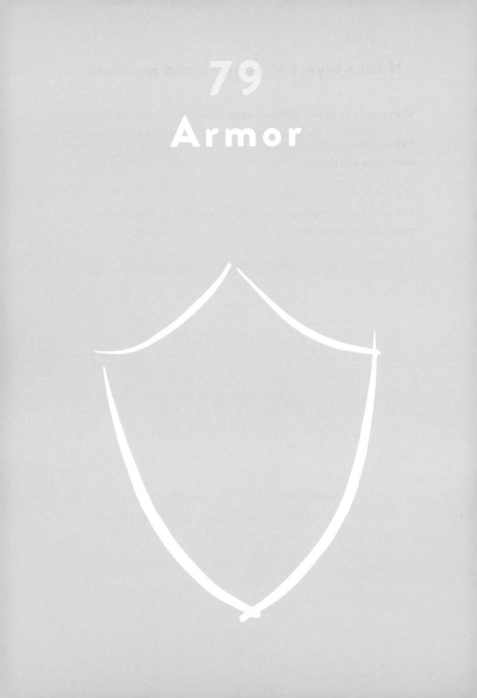

79
Armor

Notice layers of tension and protection.

Can you feel any holding in your body?

Where does tension accumulate? Can you affiliate this armor with past experiences?

Do layers of tension physically bind you to the past? Consider the process of shedding armor. How might you move in order to release and let go?

Help your body catch up to the present moment.

"You translate everything, whether physical, mental, or spiritual, into muscular tension."—F. M. Alexander

80
Acceptance

With awareness, accept your body.

Connect with the aspects of your body that you would like to change or improve. Feel your compromised and stressed parts.

Slow down your breathing. Give yourself permission to pause and be OK with your body right now.

With full awareness of the challenges and discomforts, invite peace and acceptance.

"The curious paradox is that when I accept myself just as I am, then I change."—Carl Rogers

81
Pain as a
Teacher

There's a hidden gift inside your pain.

Think of an episode of pain or discomfort you've experienced in your body.

Be with the sensations of the memory and the story.

What gift emerged from the experience? What did you learn?

"Man needs difficulties; they are necessary for health."
—Carl Jung

82
Normal
Function

Strange function can feel normal; normal function can feel strange.

In a standing position, bring your attention to the inner landscape of your body.

Notice the familiarity of your body's current state. Dysfunction may feel "normal" if it's habitual.

As you realign and restore healthy movement patterns, do these "normal" kinesthetic patterns feel alien to you?

Though it is unfamiliar at first, your body will adjust to this more normal state of normality.

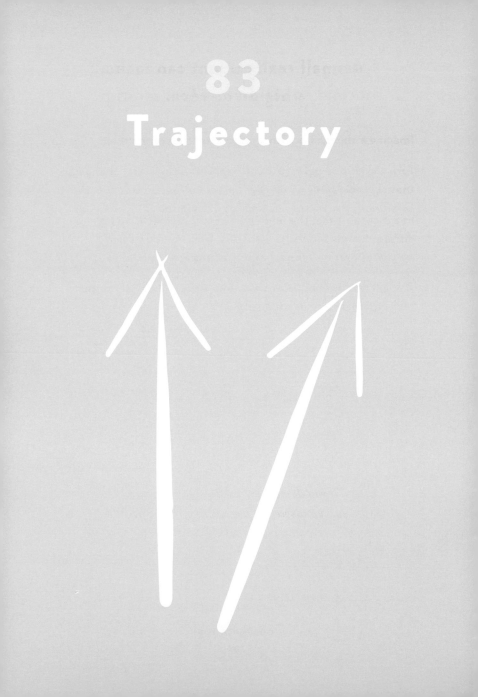

83

Trajectory

A small realignment can make a big difference.

Imagine a ship at sea with a particular trajectory.

Turn the ship to point just two degrees to the right, changing the trajectory.

In a month's time, the ending place will be much, much different.

"If you do not change direction, you may end up where you are heading."—Lao Tzu

84
Neutrality

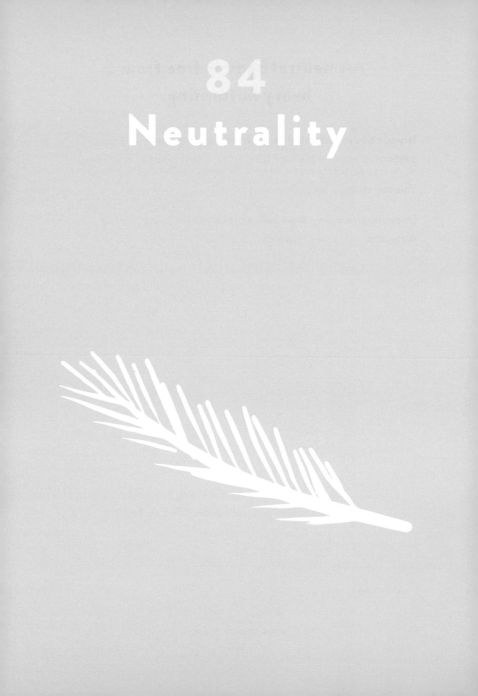

A neutral body is free from heavy patterning.

Is your body patterned in a particular direction? Are you patterned toward biking? Sitting at a desk? Yoga? Inactivity?

You are shaped by your repetitive habits.

Imagine unwinding your patterns into a more neutral state. A neutral body has more choice.

85
Current to Health

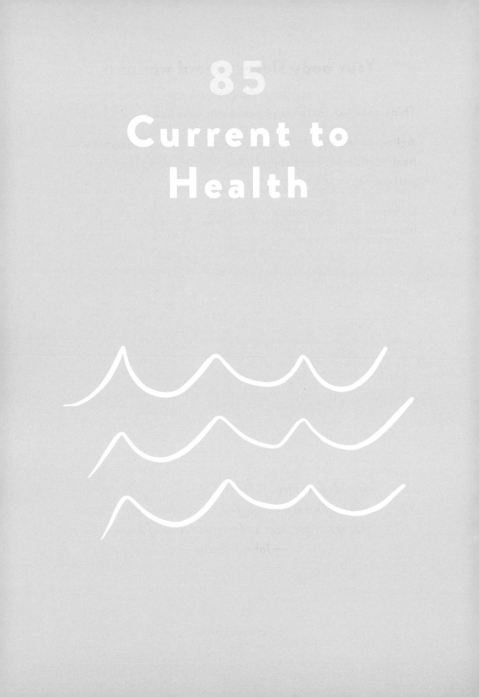

Your body flows toward wellness.

Think about an instance of healing in your body.

Acknowledge your body's capacity and innate tendency to heal itself. Even amid aberrations, injuries, and suboptimal patterning, your body is tethered to health.

Contemplate your body's inclination toward and aptitude for homeostasis.

"Your body fixes itself. A big part of this is an idea called homeostasis, which is a wonderfully intricate array of functions that repair the wear and tear and stress of living."
—John J. Ratey

86
Not-Doing

Sometimes, do nothing.

Lie down on your back. Adjust your flesh so that your whole back feels long. Let your awareness fill the inner landscape of your body.

Slow down. Let go. And then let go of letting go.

Cease all doing.

"Practice not-doing, and everything will fall into place."—Tao Te Ching

87

Absorption

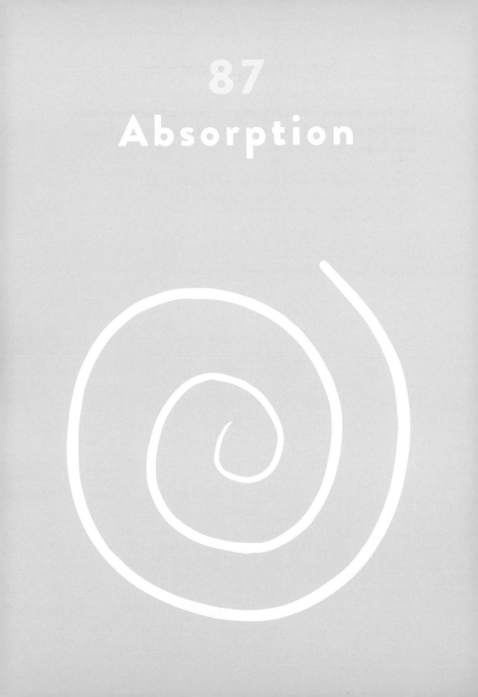

Drop in fully.

Lie down on your back. Adjust your flesh so that your whole back feels long. Let your awareness fill the inner landscape of your body.

Bring your attention to your breathing. Let your next exhale be very slow, smooth, and complete. Pause. Take a couple of normal breaths.

Let your next exhale be even slower and smoother. Pause.

Continue to practice these gradual, complete exhalations.

Surrender to the experience.

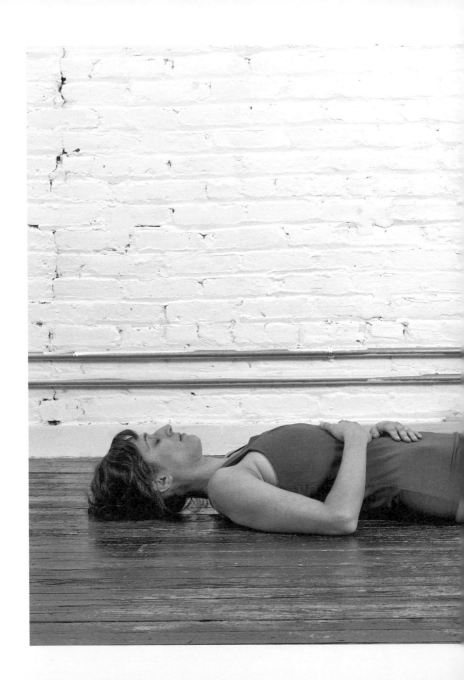

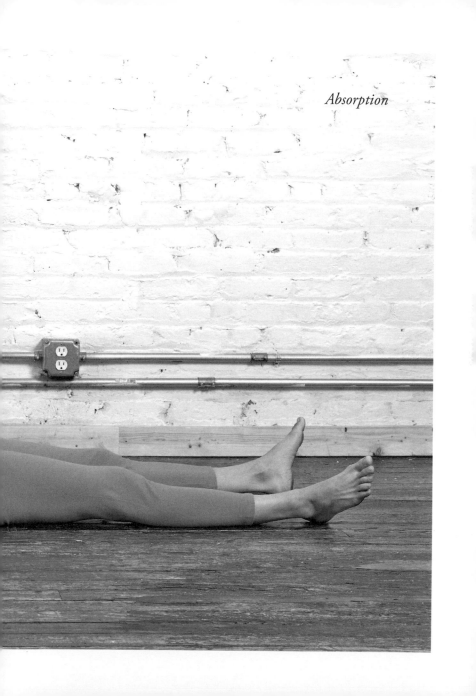

Absorption

88
Gestation

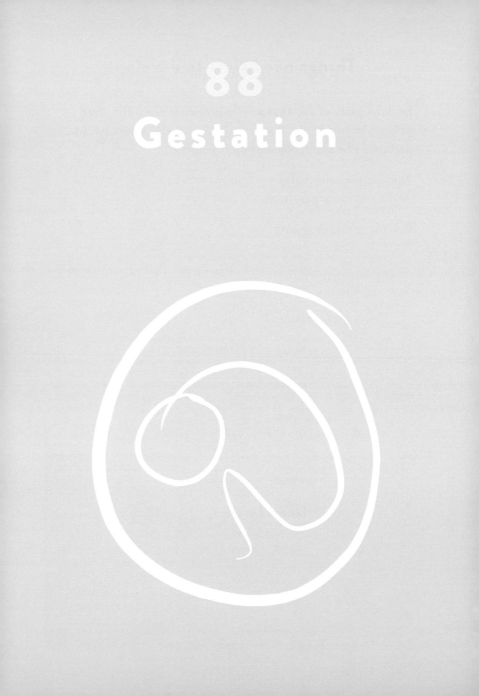

Things need time to develop.

Feel the parts of you that are "in process"—the unfinished projects in your body, the unhealed injuries, the unresolved patterns, the unestablished better habits.

Acknowledge this unfinished business in your body as parts in development, in gestation.

Relax into this moment.

"I need

more of the night before I open

eyes and heart

to illumination. I must still

grow in the dark like a root

not ready, not ready at all."

—Denise Levertov

89
Solitude

You, alone, live in your body.

Find a comfortable position. Bring your attention to the inner landscape of your body.

Welcome yourself to your embodied solitude, a place for rich learning.

Let your imagination open as you dive deeper on this solo journey inward. What sensations arise? What images? Colors? Sounds? Shapes? Memories? Desires?

"I never found the companion that was so companionable as solitude."—Henry David Thoreau

90
Wild Body

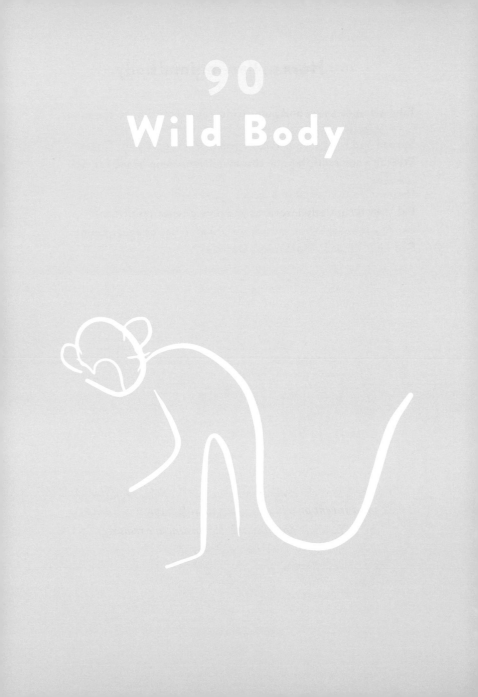

Humans are animals.

Take off your shoes and go outside.

Spread and wiggle your toes. Spread and wiggle your fingers.
Stretch your arms, legs, and spine. Take a deep breath.

Remember that you are a mammal. How do you want to move?
Feel how your body interacts with the environment.

Be in your whole body.

"We must invent or reinvent a sustainable human culture by a
descent into our pre-rational, our instinctive resources."
—Thomas Berry

91
Refined Body

Evolve through conscious refinement.

Stand with your legs and feet under you for support. Bring your attention to the inner landscape of your body, the floor, and the space around you.

Create more grounding through your legs and feet. Create a gentle lift in your spine.

Create smoothness and fullness in your breathing. Create evenness in the distribution of weight in your body.

With training and awareness, we can capitalize on natural body technology.

92
Be Pieces

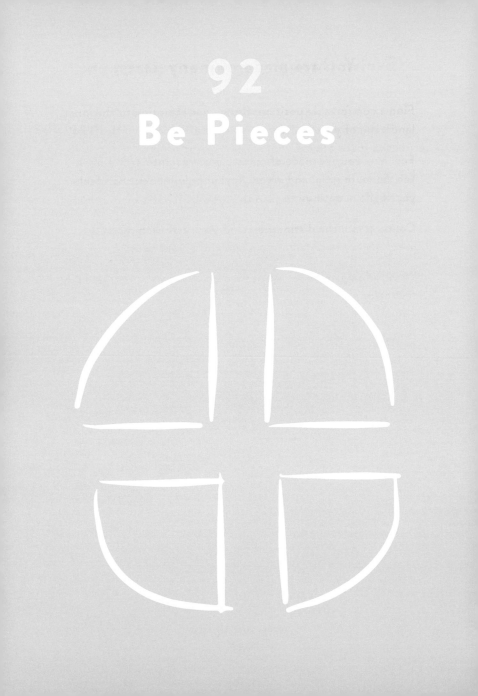

You are made of many parts.

Find a comfortable position. Bring your attention to the inner landscape of your body.

Feel how you are made of many parts. Feel into each finger, toe, bone, muscle, and organ. Feel your buttocks, then feel your belly. Continue to scan the individual parts of your body.

Contemplate the distinctness and clarity of each part.

93

Be Whole

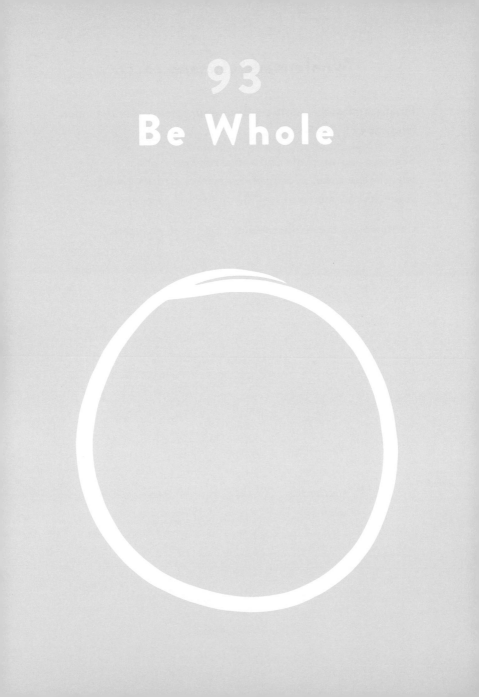

Wholeness is ever-present.

Find a comfortable position. Bring your attention to the inner landscape of your body.

Scan your entire body, from the deepest cavities to the outer edges of your skin. Feel the floor underneath you. Feel the space around you.

Contemplate your body as a vibrating, living whole.

"An effective human being is a whole that is greater than the sum of its parts."—Dr. Ida Rolf

94
Paradox

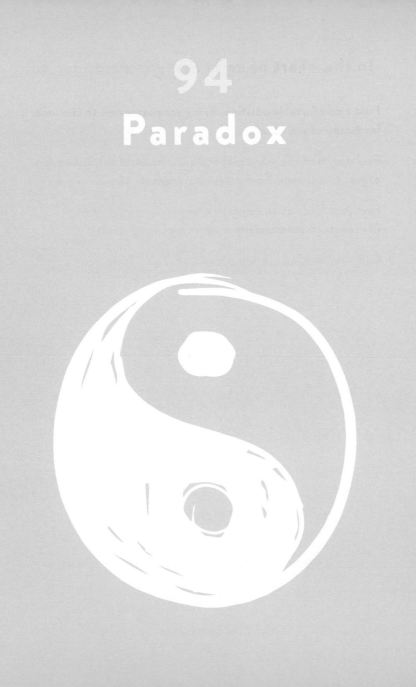

In the heart of something is its opposite.

Find a comfortable position. Bring your attention to the inner landscape of your body.

Feel your body as many pieces. In the heart of this collection of pieces is their unifying interdependence.

Feel your body as an integrated whole. In the heart of this wholeness there are many distinct pieces.

Can you think of another paradox that you embody?

95
Bodymind

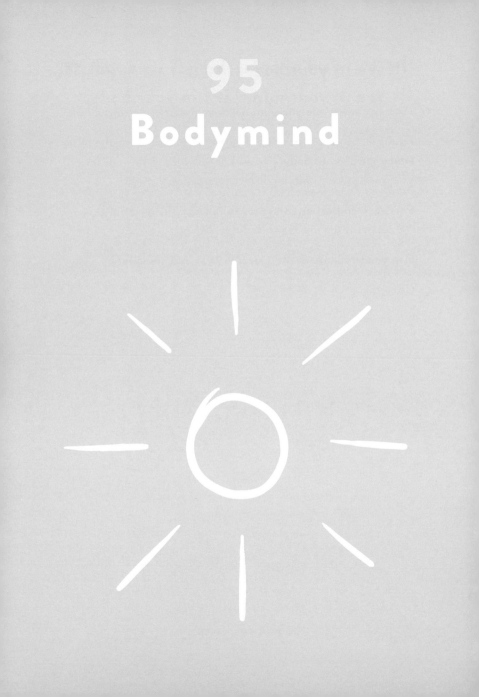

If it's in your body, it's in your mind; if it's in your mind, it's in your body.

Find a comfortable position. Bring your attention to the inner landscape of your body.

For a moment, make a tight fist with your left hand. Visualize a spark in your brain as you do that action.

Next, tune in to a personal desire. Where does this desire live in your body?

Contemplate your brain-body.

"A brain without a body could not think."
—Moshe Feldenkrais

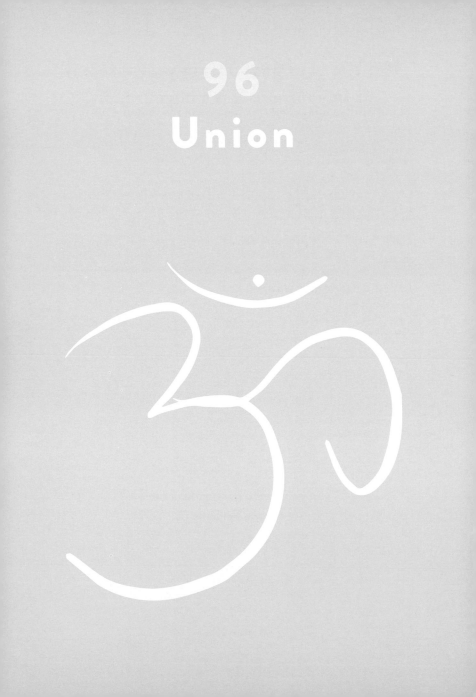

96
Union

Join opposites.

Stand with your legs and feet under you for support. As you inhale, lift your arms out to the sides and up overhead. As you exhale, lower your arms out to the sides and down.

Add another dimension. As you inhale and reach the arms up, simultaneously get grounded in your legs and feet. As you exhale and lower your arms, simultaneously lift your spine and expand your rib cage.

Continue. Get grounded as you inhale because the inhale naturally has expansion; expand as you exhale because the exhale naturally has grounding.

Observe the effects.

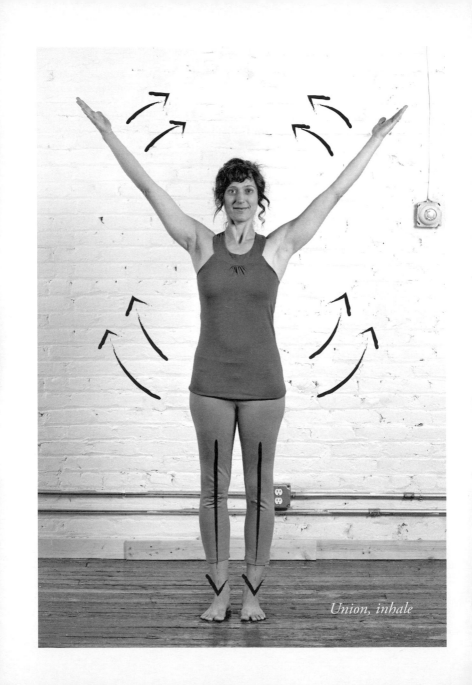

Union, inhale

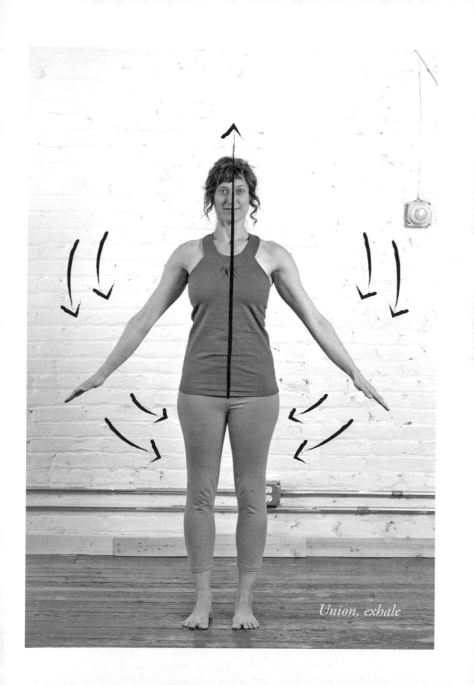

Union, exhale

97
Kinesthetic Longing

Seek your body's poetry.

Find a comfortable position. Bring your attention to the inner landscape of your body.

What form does your body want to take? What would be aesthetically fulfilling? How does your body want to move? What would be kinesthetically fulfilling?

Acknowledge your physical longings. Let them motivate and guide you.

"The symbols of the self arise in the depths of the body."
—Carl Jung

98
Bewilderment

Not knowing will serve you well.

Find a comfortable position. Bring your attention to the inner landscape of your body.

Feel into the mystery and complexity of your body and life.

Allow yourself to wonder freely without manufacturing answers.

"The most beautiful thing we can experience is the mysterious. It is the source of all true art and science."—**Albert Einstein**

99

Order Creates Freedom

Constraints can be more liberating than limiting.

Establish the following two constraints for a movement activity. Be on your hands and knees. Explore spinal movement.

Within these clear parameters, a world of creative possibilities opens up.

Apply this teaching to the movement of your body. Within the parameters of sound structure, your body can move with ease.

100
Human
Potential

You have a potential worth pursuing.

What is your unique flair?

What animates you? What is your way of moving through the world?

What will you do with your time here on Earth?

"There is nothing in a caterpillar that tells you it's going to be a butterfly."—R. Buckminster Fuller

Basic Body Landmarks

The following images will help you locate and visualize parts of your body.

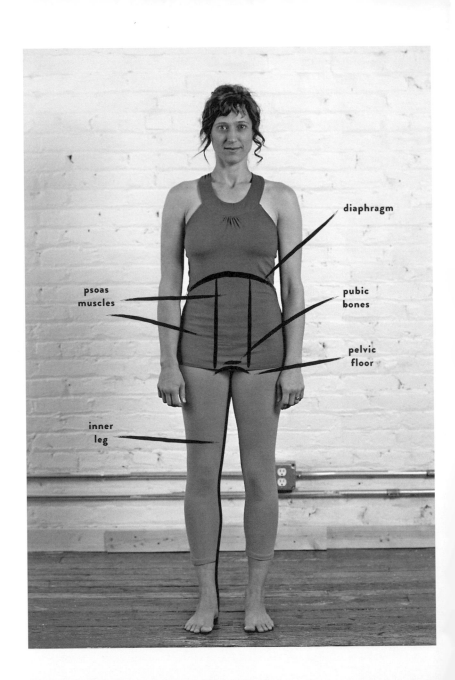

diaphragm

psoas
muscles

pubic
bones

pelvic
floor

inner
leg

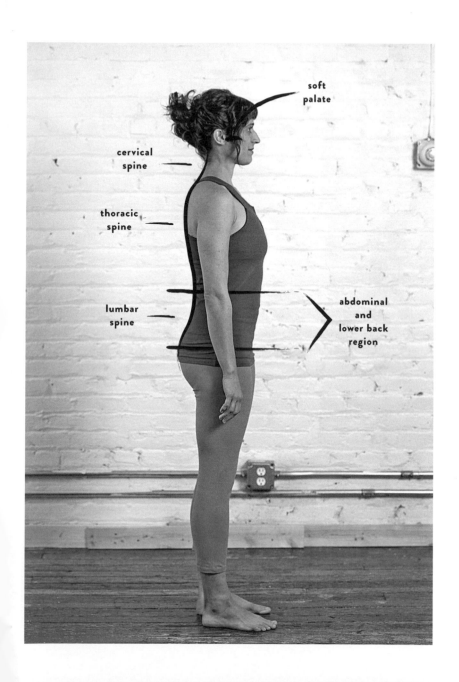

soft palate

cervical spine

thoracic spine

lumbar spine

abdominal and lower back region

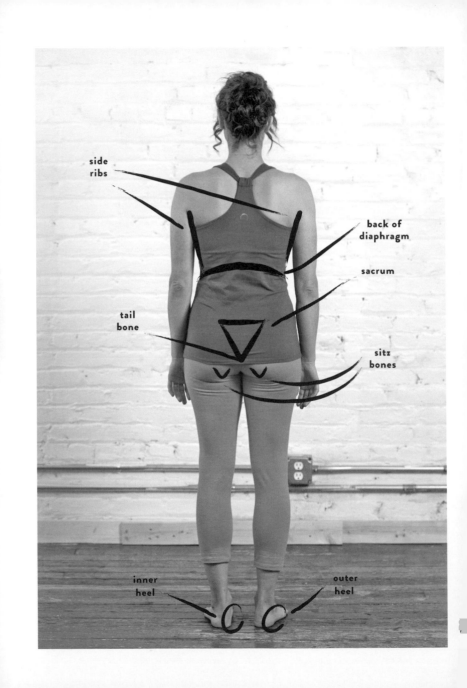

side
ribs

back of
diaphragm

sacrum

tail
bone

sitz
bones

inner
heel

outer
heel

Glossary

abdominal and lower back region – the body segment between the rib cage and the pelvis

adaptive patterns – ways the body changes in response to life experiences

Alexander Technique – a method developed by F. M. Alexander for transforming posture and body habits through awareness

cervical spine – the seven vertebrae in the neck

constitutional tendencies – patterns in musculature and alignment defined by genetic predispositions and deeply ingrained adaptive patterns

core – the deepest layers of muscles in the body, which work together to stabilize the spine and pelvis, essential for balance and coordination

diaphragm – the dome-shaped breathing muscle at the base of the rib cage

fascia – the complex web of connective tissue that envelops, divides, and connects all of the structures in the body

Feldenkrais Method – a movement-based education method, developed by Moshe Feldenkrais to improve the body-brain connection and promote personal growth

inner heel – the inner half of the weight-bearing surface of the heel

inner leg – the inner surface of the leg from the ankle to the upper thigh

internal intercostal muscles – the deepest layer of muscles, located in between the ribs, involved in the mechanics of breathing

Iyengar Yoga – a yoga method, founded by B. K. S. Iyengar and taught worldwide, known for its precision, depth, and transformative power

kinesthetic – related to movement

lumbar spine – the five vertebrae in the lower back

outer heel – the outer half of the weight-bearing surface of the heel

pelvic floor – the layered muscles at the base of the pelvis, bordered by the sitz bones, pubic bones, and tailbone

proprioception – the sense of knowing where one's own body is in space

psoas muscles – two deep abdominal muscles (right and left) that run along the front of the lumbar spine, behind the organs, and in front of the pelvis, and finally join with the upper inner thigh bones deep in the groin region

pubic bones – two bones that meet at the front of the pelvis right above the genitals

Rolf, Ida P. – scientist, healer, and founder of Structural Integration

sacrum – the triangular bone at the base of the spinal column, between the right and left pelvic bones

side ribs – the sides of the ribs, below the underarms

sitz bones – the bones at the bottom of the pelvis that are felt under the right and left buttocks and that take the body's weight when a person sits (also known as the ischial tuberosities)

soft palate – the fleshy, flexible area behind the roof of the mouth

Structural Integration – the bodywork method founded by Dr. Ida Rolf that aims to improve the body's structure and function through hands-on manipulation and movement education

tailbone – the bottom tip of the sacrum (also known as the coccyx)

thoracic spine – the twelve vertebrae in the upper and middle back

Further Reading

STRUCTURAL INTEGRATION

Bond, Mary. *The New Rules of Posture: How to Sit, Stand, and Move in the Modern World*. Rochester, VT: Healing Arts Press, 2007.

Rolf, Ida. *Rolfing and Physical Reality*. Edited by Rosemary Feitis. Rochester, VT: Healing Arts Press, 1990.

Sise, Betsy. *The Rolfing Experience: Integration in the Gravity Field*. Chino Valley, AZ: Hohm Press, 2005.

YOGA

Lasater, Judith. *Relax and Renew: Restful Yoga for Stressful Times*. Berkeley, CA: Shambhala, 2005.

Mehta, Silva, Mira Mehta, and Shyam Mehta. *Yoga: the Iyengar Way*. New York: Alfred A. Knopf, 1990.

RELATED METHODOLOGIES

Bowman, Katy Ann. *Move Your DNA: Restore Your Health Through Natural Movement*. Carlsborg, WA: Propriometrics Press, 2014.

Feldenkrais, Moshe. *Awareness Through Movement: Easy-to-Do Health Exercises to Improve Your Posture, Vision, Imagination, and Personal Awareness*. New York: HarperCollins, 1990.

Forencich, Frank. *Exuberant Animal: The Power of Health, Play and Joyful Movement*. Bloomington, IN: AuthorHouse, 2006.

Gokhale, Esther. *8 Steps to a Pain-Free Back: Natural Posture Solutions for Pain in the Back, Neck, Shoulder, Hip, Knee, and Foot*. Stanford, CA: Pendo Press, 2008.

Koch, Liz. *Core Awareness: Enhancing Yoga, Pilates, Exercise, and Dance*. Berkeley, CA: North Atlantic Books, 2012.

Acknowledgments

Thank you to Matthew Lore for seeing the virtue in this project, to Batya Rosenblum for her invaluable editing and contributions, and to the whole team at The Experiment for bringing this book to life. Thank you to the Park Slope Food Coop for my fortuitous encounter with Matthew Lore. Thank you to Hyde for the beautiful organic clothing in the book's photographs. Thank you to Sarah Toatley for her superb eye and advice, and to my brother Aaron Streiter for co-creating the Stack Your Bones app and helping to redefine the identity of *Stack Your Bones*.

Thank you to the Guild for Structural Integration and to Emmett Hutchins, Structural Integration master, for his unforgettable elegance and wisdom. Thank you to Kimberly Johnson for introducing me to Structural Integration and changing my life's path. Thank you to my teachers and mentors, especially Cyndi Lee, Tom Gillette, Lara Warren, Hugh Millard, Matt Dreyfus, Willy Kaye, Kathy Wahlund, Mary Abrams, and Bridgit Dengel Gaspard.

Thank you to my colleagues in body-oriented professions, especially James Counsellor, Lela Beem, Nick Beem, Rachel Feinberg, Sarah Chase, Sara Nolan, Livia Cohen-Shapiro, Pam Samuelson, Bonnie Crellin, and Jessa Zinn for their encouragement, support, and admirable work.

Thank you to all of my clients who are my teachers. Thank you to my son Myles for inspiring me infinitely and teaching me about being human. And most of all, thank you to my husband Eric Fraser, for supporting me during the creation process of this book (and beyond) and for continually showing me the light.

Permissions Acknowledgments

About the Author

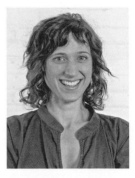

RUTHIE FRASER is a Structural Integration practitioner, yoga teacher, and movement guide. A graduate of the Guild for Structural Integration, Ruthie has been in private practice in New York City since 2007 and currently runs the Stack Your Bones Studio in Brooklyn. Ruthie has worked with hundreds of clients, blending Structural Integration with her developing movement methodology. She has trained extensively in yoga with many master teachers and has taught thousands of classes in the United States and abroad. She is also a lifelong dancer, a long-time Iyengar Yoga student, and a budding Voice Dialogue facilitator. Ruthie lives in New York, splitting her time between Brooklyn and Hudson.